Herbal Re Self Care for Common Colds, Flu, Virus

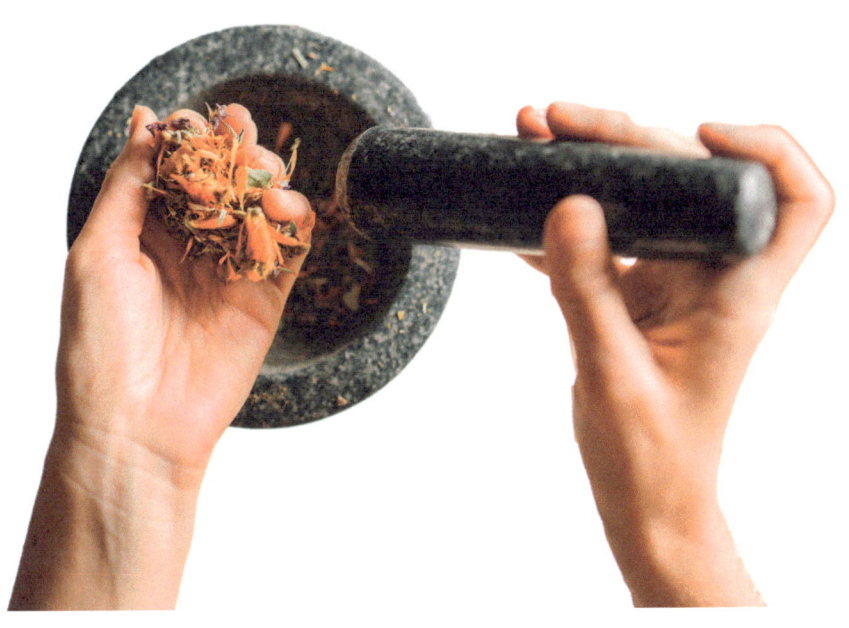

Anna Sangemino

TABLE OF CONTENTS

Foreword 5

Introduction 7

Alcohol Suggestions for Making Tinctures 11

Chapter 1. Diaphoretic Herbs 13

    Preparation & Dosage 14

    Diaphoretic Food and Recipes 29

Chapter 2. Demulcent Herbs 33

    Preparation & Dosage 33

    Demulcent Food & Dosage 42

Chapter 3. Expectorant Herbs 49

    Preparation & Dosage 50

    Expectorant Food & Recipes 64

Chapter 4. Antiviral Herbs (Antimicrobial) 69

    Preparation & Dosage 70

    Antiviral Food & Recipes 90

Chapter 5. Astringent Herbs 93

    Preparation & Dosage 94

    Astringent Food & Recipes 128

Chapter 6. Carminative Herbs 131

    Preparation & Dosage 131

    Carminative Foods and Recipes 143

Chapter 7. Adaptogen Herbs 147
    Preparation & Dosage 149
    Rejuvenating Adaptogen Foods and Recipes 156
Chapter 8. Sedative Herbs 161
    Preparation and dosage 162
    Food and Recipes with Calming Effects 170
Chapter 9. Bitter Stomachic Herbs 173
    Preparation & Dosage 174
    Food and Recipes That Aid Digestion 186
Chapter 10. Tonic Herbs 195
    Preparation & Dosage 197
    Tonic Foods and Recipes 207
Conclusion 211

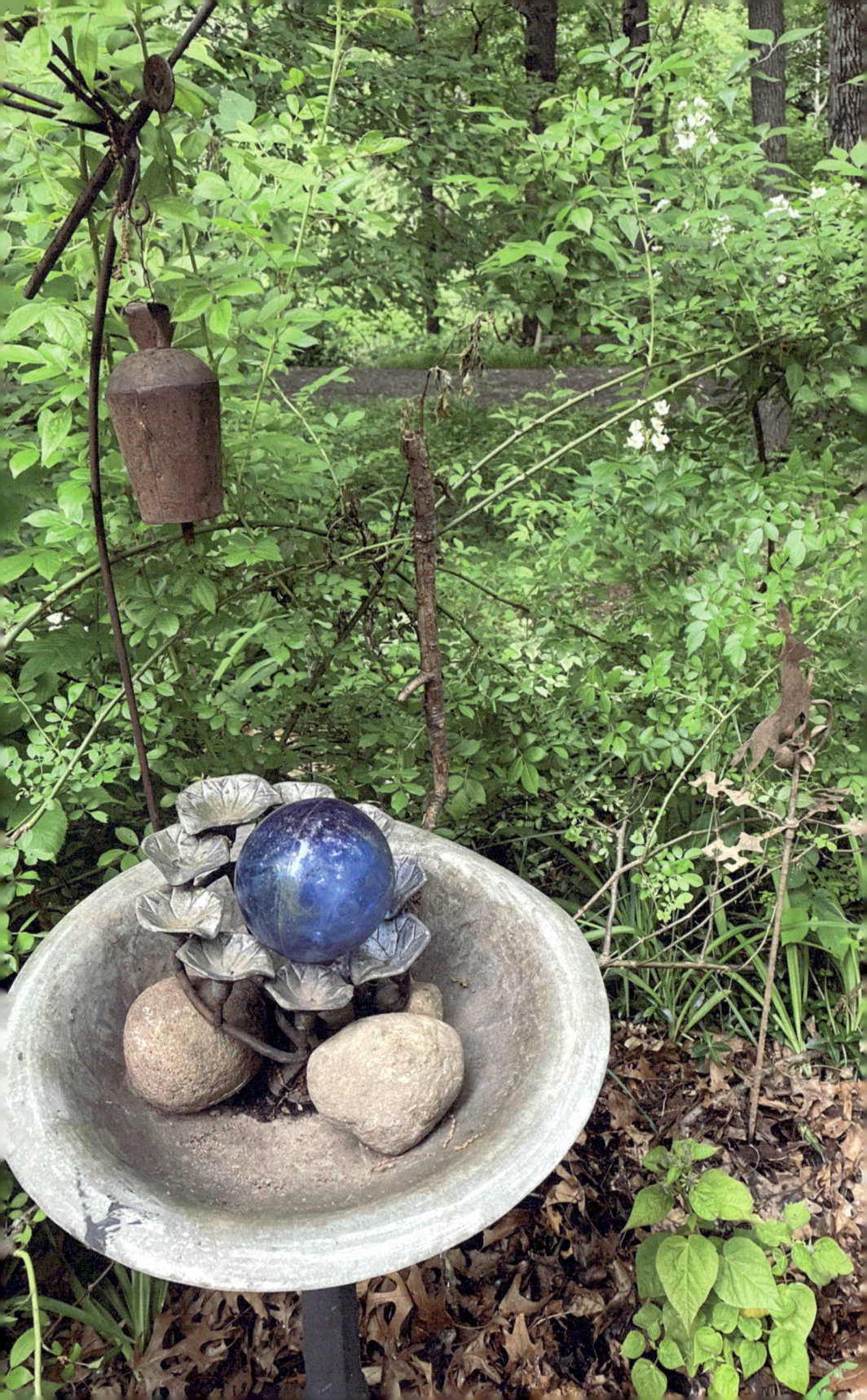

FOREWORD

Herbal medicine has been used for thousands of years across cultures all around the world to treat various illnesses and health conditions. Throughout history, herbal remedies have continuously evolved and become increasingly refined as plant preparation and methods have been revealed and discovered.

Today, herbal remedies are widely recognized as an alternative approach to conventional medicine. Many people turn to herbal remedies and even learn how to make them at home for treating acute illnesses such as colds, flu, and viruses as well as chronic health conditions such as allergies and digestive issues. This approach involves knowing the herbal actions and properties that can address underlying imbalances and support the body's natural healing processes.

In recent years, there has been a rapidly growing interest in the use of herbs for treating viruses, particularly in light of COVID-19. With limited conventional treatment options available, many people have turned to herbs and botanicals as a natural and potentially effective way to support their immune system and fight off viruses.

One major advantage of herbal medicine is that it often results in fewer side effects compared to conventional drugs. This is because herbs and botanicals contain a complex mix of active compounds that work together to produce therapeutic effects. When used in the right way and in the right amounts, these compounds can help to alleviate symptoms and promote healing without causing adverse effects.

By the end of this book, readers will have a comprehensive understanding of the benefits of herbal remedies and their role in treating viruses and enjoy a variety of practical tips, recipes, and herbal preparations for self-care.

INTRODUCTION

When one begins to explore the world of herbal medicine, many questions come to mind. What part of the herb do I use—the root, leaf, or flower? Do I need tea, a tincture, or both for my illness? How much should I use to make my own remedy, how much should I use, and how often should I take it? Which herb should I consider using to address specific symptoms? How do I combine herbs with proper nutrition during an illness? This book aims to answer these questions and provide readers with an in-depth understanding of how herbs work to treat the common cold, the flu, and other viruses. Food is medicine, and so you will see recipes and beverages included in each chapter to support herbal actions, bring comfort, and alleviate symptoms.

We will explore the potential pathways of viruses, how they affect the body, and how the herbal actions support the immune system in fighting off infections. All of the questions I always had in the early days of my herbal studies; I have answered here. For instance, is tea more effective than a tincture for a sore throat? What is the correct dosage for children? Can I take an herbal extract with confidence that it will help me get better? Will this meal weaken my immune system or elevate my symptoms, making my condition worse? What should I eat, that will help me feel better?

In this book, each chapter presents the herbal actions, botanical topical applications, and foods to eat that will effectively support the immune system while the illness runs its course. These elements are presented in a recipe format to be prepared for treating viruses in a variety of ways. Some of the most common preparation methods include teas, tinctures, essential oils for topical applications, and food recipes. Each herbal action has its own specific antidote for the related symptoms, and the best preparation method will be a choice you can make for your own self-care and spiritual well-being.

The physical illnesses and symptoms caused by each virus are described in each chapter so that you can be fully informed and choose and prepare the best herbal solutions for you with confidence. In addition, the included food recipes support the herbal actions and provide comfort for the disease you are feeling. The foods chosen for each chapter support the herbal actions and the healing processes described in each chapter for the desired therapeutic effect.

After gaining some knowledge and experience, you can also make your own blends by combining different herbs that address your symptoms from each category. You may find that a single herb addresses more than one symptom, or you may want to make a stronger concoction by adding the herbs and tinctures together to your tea or food.

For example, teas are a popular and simple way to use herbs for viral infections. Herbal infusions (e.g., tea) are easy enough to make by steeping fresh or dried herbs in hot water. Teas are often prepared for respiratory infections caused by viruses, such as colds, the flu, and viral infections. You can add tea to your smoothies and main dishes. You can also add a tincture to a cup of herbal tea for a stronger remedy.

The essential oils discussed in this book are intended for topical use or for aromatherapy by being added to a diffuser to purify the air from airborne pathogens. For aromatherapy, essential oils are often used as steam vapors or a cold-diffused vapor and inhaled for the beneficial effects of their minute molecular structure. When used topically, they are blended with carrier oils and rubbed over the skin where the underlying condition is. You can also breathe in their aroma as the essential oils filter through the air for your comfort, health, and well-being.

In addition to herbs and botanicals, nutrition also plays a vital role in supporting the immune system during a viral infection. Eating a diet of whole foods consisting of fruits, vegetables, plants from the sea (seaweed), and whole grains can provide the body with the nutrients it needs to adequately fight off infections as well as support herbal actions.

Protein is essential for the proper functioning of the immune system. Antibodies, a protective protein, play a crucial role in fighting infections. Plant compounds are proteins, and lean proteins such as fish, chicken, turkey, and tofu can help provide the body with the necessary building blocks to create antibodies and other immune system components. Additionally, protein helps repair and regenerate the body's tissues, including those damaged by infection, and can help maintain muscle mass, which is important for overall health and physical strength during illness. Certain supplements such as vitamin C, D, and zinc are particularly important for immune function and can be taken to support healing as well.

The use of herbal remedies for treating viruses offers a safe and effective alternative to conventional treatments. By understanding the role of herbs, botanicals, and a proper diet in supporting the immune system and making slight changes to one's lifestyle, individuals can take an active role in prioritizing their health and promoting healing in a natural and holistic way.

ALCOHOL SUGGESTIONS FOR MAKING TINCTURES

40% to 50% alcohol by volume	67.5% to 70% alcohol by volume	85% to 95% alcohol by volume
80- to 100-proof alcohol (usually vodka)	A blend of approx. 50% 80-proof vodka and 50% 151- to 190-proof grain alcohol	190-proof grain alcohol (also known as Everclear or moonshine)
Easily available and most commonly used.	For efficient extraction of aromatic properties and volatile compounds.	While overkill for most herbs in tincturing, it is an efficient solvent option for extracting from gums and resins.
Suitable for most dried herbs or fresh herbs that are set to wilt for a day before tincturing.	A great match for lemon balm, berries, turmeric, and ginger aromatic roots.	More efficiently extracts the essential oils and aromatic compounds that are harder to extract.
Pro: Aids in the efficient extraction of water-soluble properties as well.	Pro: The blended higher-strength alcohol will extract more of the plant fluids.	Con: The high alcohol strength can produce results that are literally hard to swallow.

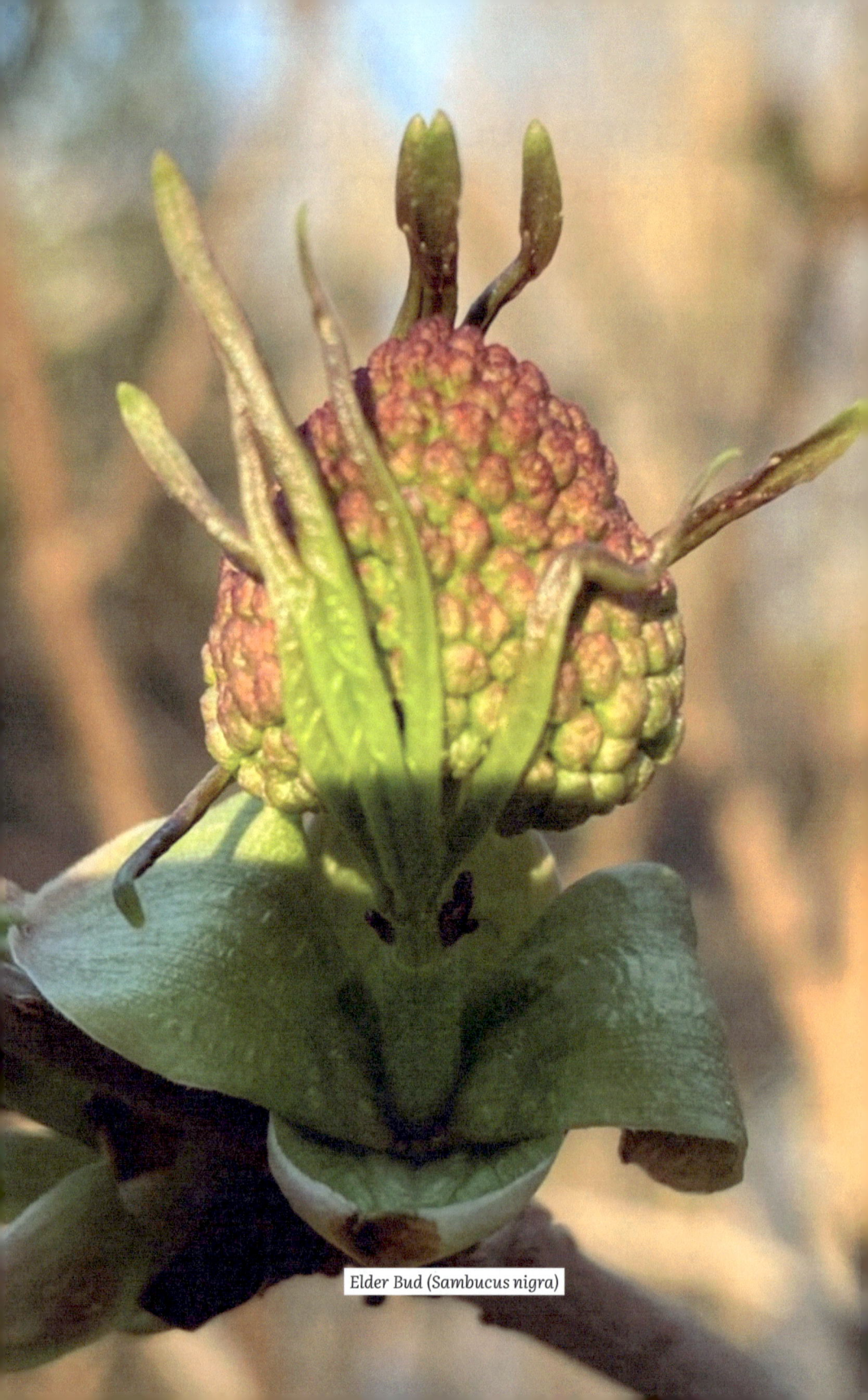
Elder Bud (Sambucus nigra)

CHAPTER 1.
DIAPHORETIC HERBS

Herbal diaphoretics are a group of herbs that promote sweating and increase overall body temperature. Sweating helps to eliminate toxins from the body while also cooling the body down in cases of fever or overheating. Diaphoretics work by dilating the blood vessels close to the skin's surface, allowing heat to escape by triggering the sweat glands to produce sweat. Many diaphoretic herbs are also antimicrobial and immune stimulating, making them helpful for fighting off infections such as colds, flu, and viruses.

A. Ginger (Zingiber officinale)
B. Yarrow (Achillea millefolium)
C. Elderflower (Sambucus nigra)
D. Sweet basil (Ocimum basilicum)
E. Holy basil (Ocimum tenuiflorum)
F. Lemon balm (Melissa officinalis)
G. Chrysanthemum (Chrysanthemum × morifolium)
H. Bee balm (Monarda fistulosa)

Preparation methods for diaphoretic herbs can include making teas, tinctures, and using steam. It is important to use caution with diaphoretics, as they can cause dehydration if not used properly. Drink plenty of fluids and get adequate rest when using diaphoretics to support the immune system so that the virus does not manifest deeper into the circulatory system.

Preparation & Dosage

Ginger (Zingiber officinale)

Ginger can be added to food recipes fresh, dried, or as a tea or tincture. To produce a sweat or break a fever, add ginger to a soup, make a cup of ginger tea and add a ginger tincture, or drink ginger tea with fresh or dried ginger. Afterwards, wrap up in cotton or flannel pajamas, go to bed, and stay covered until you have completely broken your fever by sweating. This process may protect the body from a full-fledged viral infection.

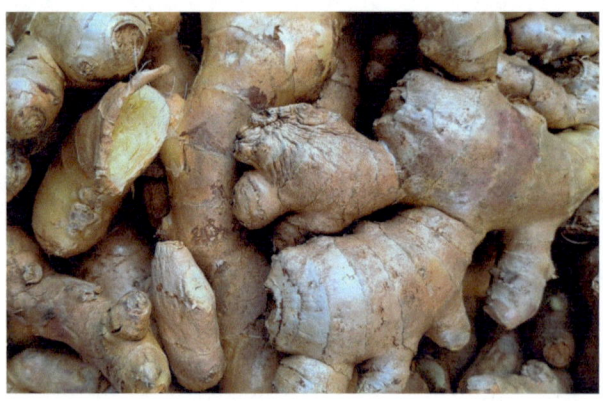

Ginger Infusion Recipe:

- Slice fresh ginger root (about 1-2 inches) OR use 2 teaspoons of dried ginger root.
- Pour a pint of simmering water over the ginger, then cover with a lid.
- Steep for 10 minutes.
- Strain.
- Add honey or maple syrup and lemon if desired.
- For a stronger tea, you can use more ginger.

Ginger Tincture Recipe:

- Chop fresh ginger root OR dried ginger root into small pieces and place into a jar.
- Pour in enough alcohol to cover, leaving space at the top.*
- Tightly seal the jar, label, date, and shake well.
- Let it steep for 2–3 months. Shake the jar weekly.
- Strain the mixture, then store it in a glass jar in a dark place.
- Take 10–20 drops diluted in a little bit of water up to three times a day as needed.
- For children, the proper amount will vary depending on their age and weight. Use 3–5 drops diluted in a small amount of juice or water up to three times a day as needed.

*For all tincture recipes, please refer to "Alcohol Suggestions for Making Tinctures" to help you decide which alcohol will work best for you.

Note: Every tincture recipe in this book can be adjusted to make a larger or smaller batch. Additionally, the strength and potency of the tincture may vary depending on the amount of alcohol used and the duration of the steeping process.

Ginger Capsule Recipe:

- You can either fill your own or purchase ginger capsules at health food stores or online. The recommended dosage is usually 500–1000 mg (about the weight of a small paper clip) of ginger powder taken up to three times a day.

Note: Always consult with a clinical herbalist or health care professional before taking herbal remedies, particularly if you have a health-related condition or are taking medication.

Yarrow (Achillea millefolium)

Yarrow supports the body's detoxification process by inducing sweat, cleansing the lymphatic system, reducing headaches, and protecting the intestines from a buildup of toxins that can leak through the gut, causing acute inflammation throughout the body.

Yarrow Infusion Recipe:

- Fill a tea ball or an infuser with fresh yarrow leaves OR use 2 teaspoons of dried yarrow leaves. Add the leaves to a mug of simmering water.
- Steep for 10 minutes.
- Add honey or maple syrup and lemon if desired.
- For a stronger tea, you can use more yarrow.

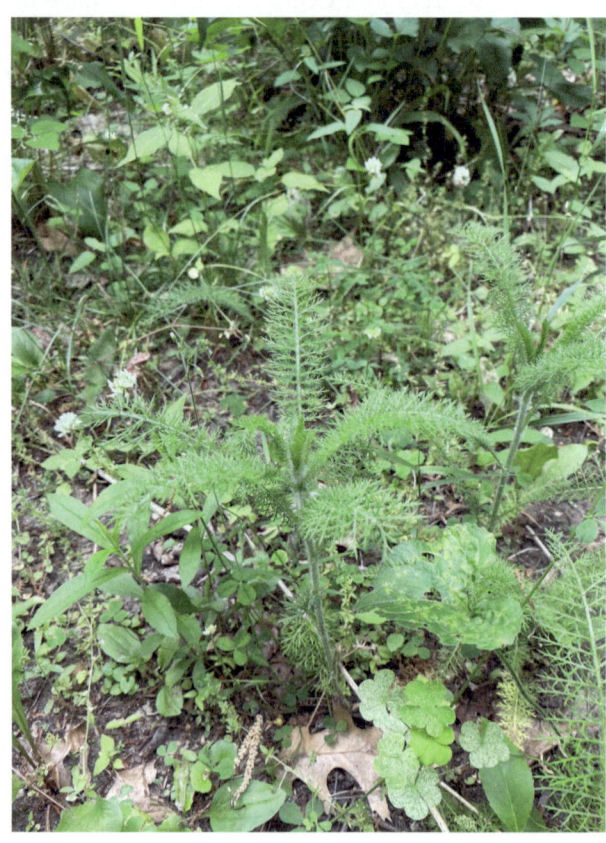

Yarrow Tincture Recipe:

- Chop fresh or dried yarrow leaves and place into a jar.
- Pour in enough alcohol to cover, leaving space at the top.*
- Tightly seal the jar, label, date, and shake well.
- Let it steep for 2–3 months. Shake the jar weekly.
- Strain the mixture, then store it in a glass jar in a dark place.
- Take 10–20 drops diluted in a little bit of water up to three times a day as needed.
- For children, the proper amount will vary depending on their age and weight. Use 3–5 drops diluted in a small amount of juice or water up to three times a day as needed.

Note: Yarrow should not be used during pregnancy or by people who are allergic to ragweed or other plants in the Asteraceae family. Always consult with a clinical herbalist or health care professional before using yarrow, particularly if you have a health condition or are taking medication.

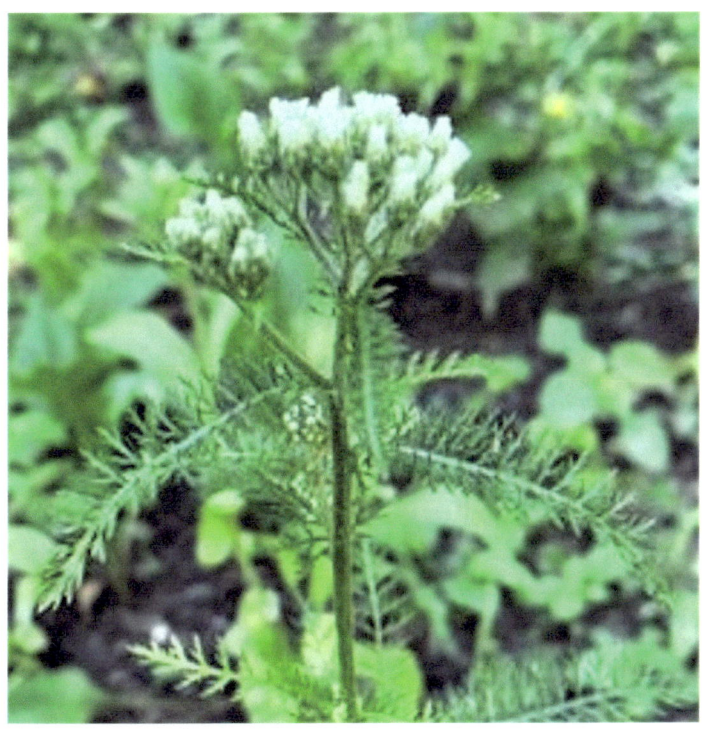

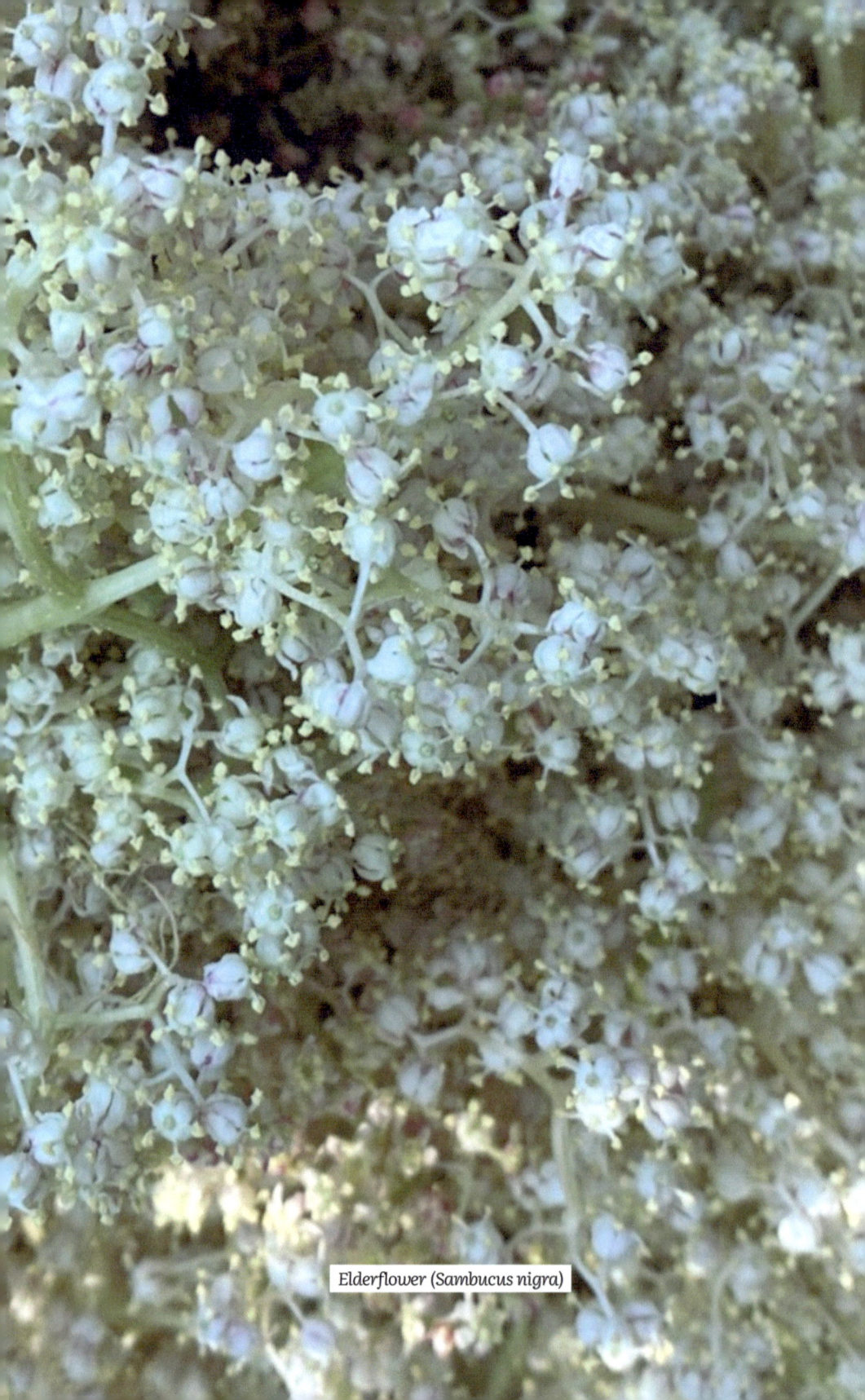
Elderflower (Sambucus nigra)

Elderflower (Sambucus nigra)

Elderflowers contain compounds that stimulate the circulatory system by increasing blood flow to the skin's surface, which increases heat loss and encourages sweating. The diaphoretic action of elderflower can help to reduce fevers and relieve symptoms of colds, flu, and viruses as well as support the immune system to fight off infections.

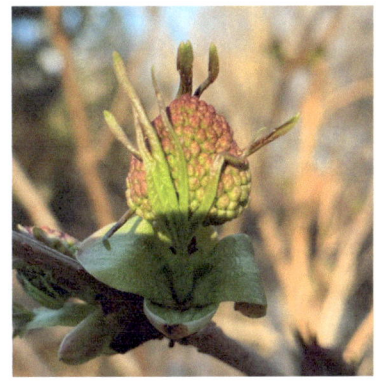

Elderflower Infusion Recipe:

- Add 4 teaspoons of fresh elderflowers OR 2 teaspoons of dried elderflowers into a mug of simmering water.
- Steep for 5–7 minutes.
- Add honey or maple syrup and lemon if desired.
- For a stronger tea, you can use more elderflowers or add 3–5 drops of elderflower tincture.
- Drink up to 3 cups a day as needed.

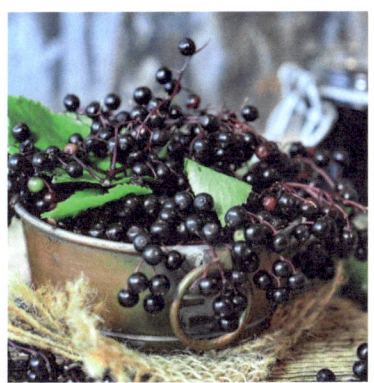

Elderflower Tincture Recipe:

- Chop fresh or dried elderflowers into pieces and place into a jar.
- Pour in enough alcohol to cover, leaving space at the top.*
- Tightly seal the jar, label, date, and shake well.
- Let it steep for 2–3 months. Shake the jar weekly.
- Strain the mixture, then store it in a glass jar in a dark place.

- Take 10–20 drops diluted in a little bit of water up to three times a day as needed.
- For children, the proper amount will vary depending on their age and weight. Use 3–5 drops diluted in a small amount of juice or water up to three times a day as needed.

Note: Elderflowers should be used with caution for individuals who are pregnant, breastfeeding, or have kidney problems. As with any herbal treatment, always consult with a clinical herbalist or a health care professional if you have a health condition or are taking medication.

Elderberry Syrup

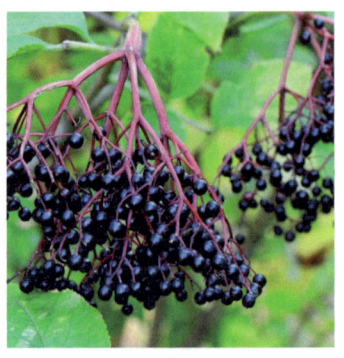

It is not typically considered a diaphoretic herb, but this syrup is a blend mixed with warming herbs that are diaphoretic. Elderberry syrup has both immune-stimulating and diaphoretic properties. It is often used to support the immune system when the person is cold, has chills, and cannot get warm enough to break a fever during viral infections such as flus and colds.

However, elderberry has been traditionally used for its diaphoretic properties in some cultures, and some preparations of elderberry may still have a mild diaphoretic effect.

Elderberry Syrup Recipe:

Ingredients:

- 1 cup elderberries (dried)
- 5 cups water

- 2 cinnamon sticks
- 1 ½ tsp powdered ginger
- ½ tsp powdered cloves
- 1 cup honey

Instructions:

- In a large pot, pour in the water, dried elderberries, cinnamon sticks, ginger, and cloves.
- Simmer for approximately 50 minutes until the liquid has evaporated by about half.
- Remove the pot from heat.
- Strain the mixture through cheesecloth, put on disposable gloves, and squeeze all the juice out of the berries.
- Add natural sweetener to taste and stir until it is well dissolved.
- Pour the syrup into a glass bottle and store it in the refrigerator for up to 2–3 months.
- Take 1 tablespoon of elderberry syrup up to four times a day as needed.
- For children, the proper amount will vary depending on their age and weight. Use 1 teaspoon diluted in a small amount of water up to four times a day as needed.

Note: Always consult with a clinical herbalist or health care professional before taking herbal remedies, particularly if you have a health-related condition or are taking medication.

Basil (Ocimum basilicum)

Basil is an aromatic herb that has traditionally been used as a diaphoretic herb for colds, flus, and viruses. Basil has warming properties that can help to promote sweating, which can aid in reducing fever and eliminating toxins from the body. Basil's antimicrobial and anti-inflammatory actions also support the body's natural healing processes during a viral infection.

Basil Infusion Recipe:

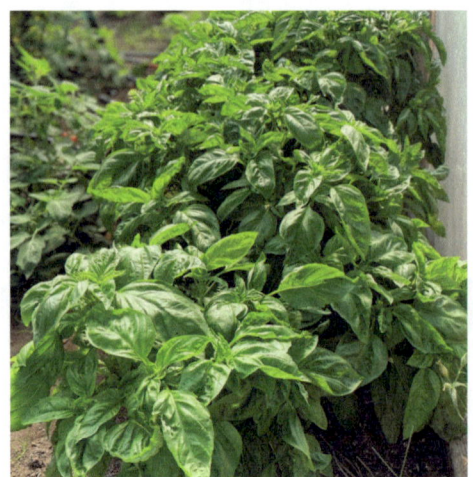

- Add 6 teaspoons of fresh basil leaves OR 3 teaspoons of dried basil leaves to a tea ball or infuser.
- Place into a mug and pour simmering water over the herbs.
- Steep for 5–7 minutes.
- Add honey or a natural sweetener if desired.
- For a stronger tea, use more basil.

Basil Tincture Recipe:

- Chop fresh basil leaves and stems into small pieces and place into a jar.
- Pour in enough alcohol to cover, leaving space at the top.*
- Tightly seal the jar, label, date, and shake well.
- Let it steep for 2–3 months. Shake the jar weekly.
- Strain the mixture, then store it in a glass jar in a dark place.
- Take 10–20 drops diluted in a little bit of water up to three times a day as needed.
- For children, the proper amount will vary depending on their age and weight. Use 3–5 drops diluted in a small amount of juice or water up to three times a day as needed.

Note: Basil is safe when used in culinary dishes, but always consult with a clinical herbalist or health care professional before taking herbal remedies, particularly if you have a health-related condition or are taking medication.

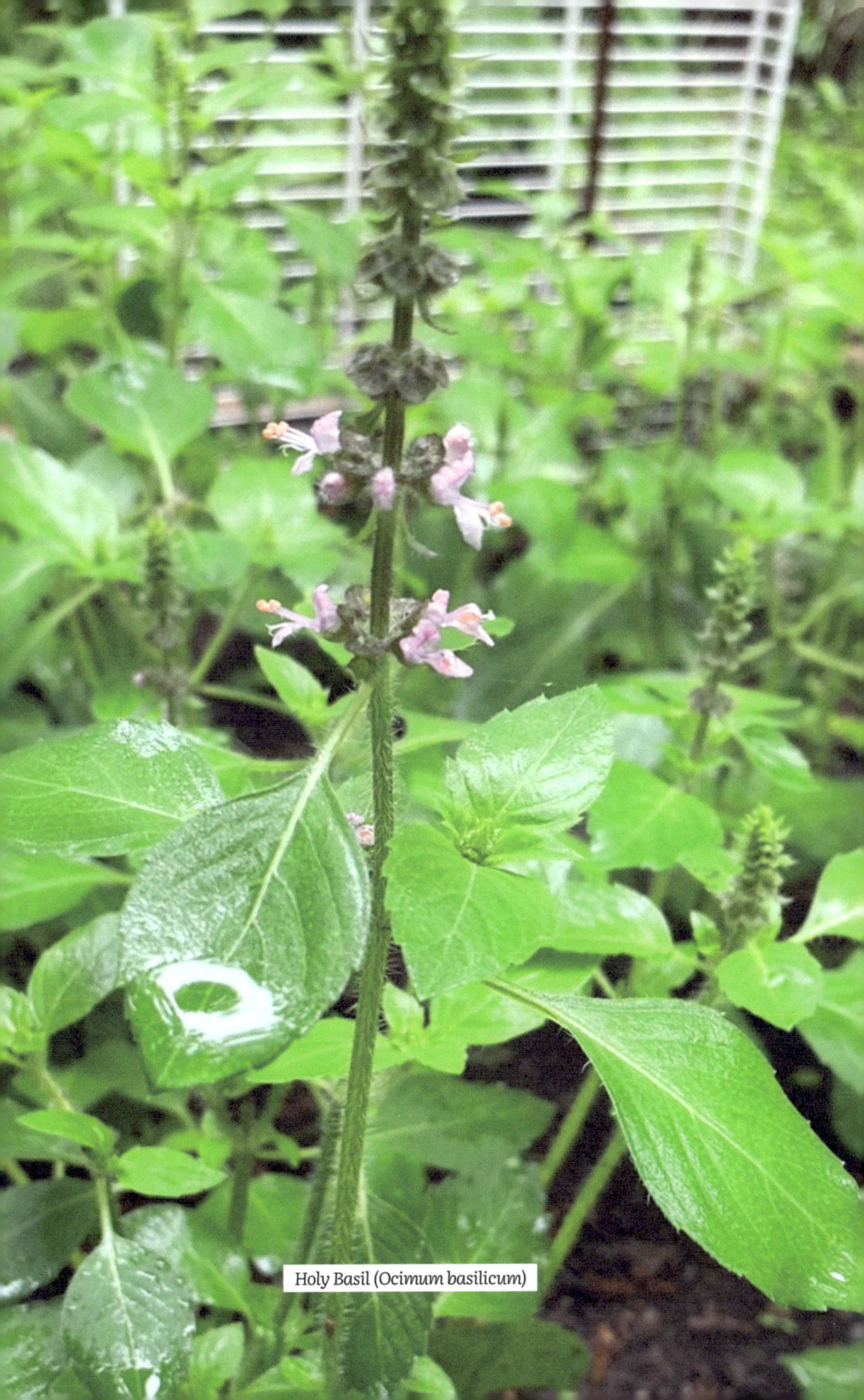

Holy Basil (Ocimum basilicum)

Holy Basil (Ocimum tenuiflorum)

Also known as tulsi, holy basil shares some similarities with sweet basil in terms of its properties as a diaphoretic herb. Both herbs contain essential oils and compounds that may help promote an increase in body temperature and sweating, which can aid in fighting off colds, flus, and viral infections.

However, holy basil is a more potent medicinal herb than sweet basil with a broader range of therapeutic properties. In addition to its diaphoretic action, holy basil is also known for its adaptogenic, anti-inflammatory, and immune-modulating effects that can further support the body during a viral infection, the common cold, or the flu.

Holy Basil Infusion Recipe:

- Add 4 teaspoons of fresh basil OR 2 teaspoons of dried leaves into an infuser.
- Place into a mug and pour simmering water over the herbs.
- Steep for 5–7 minutes.
- Drink 1–3 cups per day as needed.

Holy Basil Tincture Recipe:

- Place dried holy basil leaves into a jar.
- Pour in enough alcohol to cover, leaving space at the top.*
- Tightly seal the jar, label, date, and shake well.
- Let it steep for 2–3 months. Shake the jar weekly.
- Strain the mixture, then store it in a glass jar in a dark place.
- Take 10–15 drops diluted in a little bit of water up to three times a day as needed.
- For children, the proper amount will vary depending on their age and weight. Use 3–5 drops diluted in a small amount of juice or water up to three times a day as needed.

Note: Always consult with a clinical herbalist or health care professional before taking herbal remedies, particularly if you have a health-related condition or are taking medication.

Lemon Balm (Melissa officinalis)

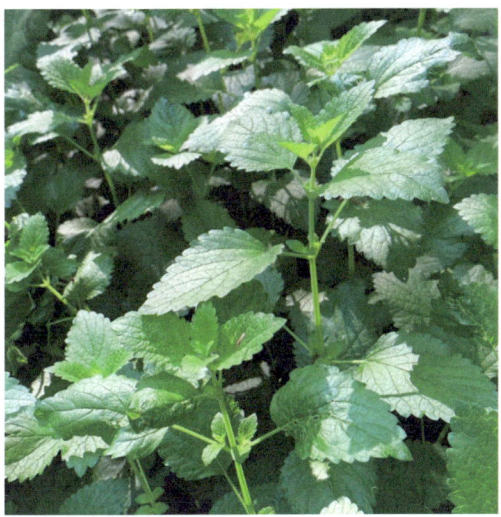

Lemon balm is known to relieve fatigue. With its calming and relaxing properties, it has a long history of use and has been known to have antiviral, antibacterial, and antioxidant effects.

As a diaphoretic, lemon balm helps to promote sweating and increase body temperature, which can help to reduce fever and fight off infections such as colds, flu, and viruses. It is also believed to have immune-boosting effects that can support the body's natural defenses against viruses and other pathogens.

Lemon balm contains compounds such as rosmarinic acid and eugenol that have been shown to possess antiviral activity against influenza viruses. These compounds work by disrupting the viral envelope and preventing the virus from replicating.

In addition to its diaphoretic and antiviral properties, lemon balm is also used to promote relaxation, reduce anxiety, and improve sleep.

Lemon Balm Infusion Recipe:

- Fresh leaves have more aromatic oil and are preferred here. Chop 3 tablespoons of fresh lemon balm leaves and add them to a tea ball.
- Place into a mug and pour simmering water over the herbs.
- Steep for 5–7 minutes.
- Add honey or maple syrup if desired.
- For a stronger tea, you can use more lemon balm.

Lemon Balm Tincture Recipe:

- Cut fresh lemon balm leaves and place into a jar.
- Pour in enough alcohol to cover, leaving space at the top.*
- Tightly seal the jar, label, date, and shake well.
- Let it steep for 2–3 months. Shake the jar weekly.
- Strain the mixture, then store it in a glass jar in a dark place.
- Take 10–20 drops diluted in a little bit of water up to three times a day as needed.
- For children, the proper amount will vary depending on their age and weight. Use 3–5 drops diluted in a small amount of juice or water up to three times a day as needed.

Note: Lemon balm is safe when used in culinary amounts. However, it may interact with certain medications, so always consult with a clinical herbalist or health care professional before use if you have a health condition, are taking medication, or are pregnant or breastfeeding.

Chrysanthemum (Chrysanthemum morifolium)

The chrysanthemum, also known as mum, is an effective diaphoretic due to its ability to induce sweating. It contains compounds that can dilate blood vessels, increase blood flow, and promote perspiration, which can help to reduce fever and detoxify and cool the body. Chrysanthemum is also known for its anti-inflammatory and antioxidant properties, which may enhance and support the immune system during a viral infection.

In traditional Chinese medicine (TCM), it is commonly used as an herbal remedy for respiratory infections, the common cold, flus, and viruses due to its herbal actions that support the immune system to promote lung function and relieve coughing.

Chrysanthemum Tea Recipe:

- Add 4–5 teaspoons of fresh chrysanthemum flowers OR 2–3 teaspoons of dried flowers into an infuser.
- Place into a mug and pour simmering water over the flowers.
- Steep for 5–7 minutes.
- Add honey or other herbs for flavor if desired.
- Drink 1–2 mugs a day as needed.
- For a stronger tea, use more chrysanthemum.

Note: Some individuals have experienced allergic reactions to chrysanthemum with side effects such as skin irritation or gastrointestinal upset. As with any herbal remedy, it is best to slowly increase the amount used over time and monitor your body's response. Always consult with a clinical herbalist or health care professional before taking herbal remedies, particularly if you have a health-related condition or are taking medication.

Bee Balm (Monarda fistulosa)

Bee balm, also known as Monarda fistulosa or wild bergamot, has several herbal actions. It has diaphoretic properties, meaning it can induce sweating and help regulate body temperature, that makes it useful for treating fevers and other illnesses associated with chills. It is also a mild sedative and can help promote relaxation and reduce anxiety. Finally, bee balm has carminative properties that can help relieve digestive issues such as gas and bloating. Drink the tea either cold or at room temperature for a carminative effect. For headaches caused by viral infections, drink warm or hot tea.

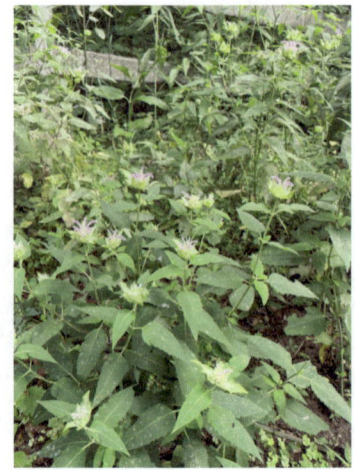

Bee balm has long been used for its antiseptic, carminative, diaphoretic, and stimulant actions. It is commonly used to treat respiratory and digestive issues.

Bee Balm Infusion Recipe:

- Add 2–3 teaspoons of dried bee balm leaves and flowers to a tea ball.
- Place into a mug and pour simmering water over the herbs.
- Steep for 5–7 minutes.
- Drink 1–3 cups a day as needed.

Bee Balm Tincture Recipe:

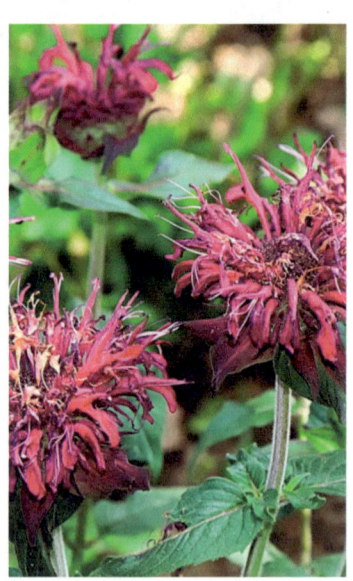

- Put fresh bee balm leaves and flowers into a jar.
- Pour in enough alcohol to cover, leaving space at the top.*
- Tightly seal the jar, label, date, and shake well.
- Let it steep for 2–3 months. Shake the jar weekly.
- Strain the mixture, then store it in a glass jar in a dark place.
- Take 10–20 drops diluted in a little bit of water up to three times a day as needed.

- For children, the proper amount will vary depending on their age and weight. Use 3–5 drops diluted in a small amount of juice or water up to three times a day as needed.

Note: Always consult with a clinical herbalist or health care professional before using bee balm, especially if you are pregnant, breastfeeding, have medical issues, or are taking any medications. Bee balm may cause allergic reactions in some individuals, particularly those who are allergic to plants in the mint family.

Diaphoretic Food and Recipes

Recipes for Meals and Snacks During the First Stage of a Cold, Flu, or Covid-19

Meals

Spicy Ginger and Turmeric Tea:

- Simmer 4 cups of water.
- Add grated ginger and grated turmeric root to the simmering water.
- Reduce heat and simmer for 10 minutes.
- Take off the heat and blend with a natural sweetener. Add lemon juice to taste.
- Strain and drink hot.

Chicken Soup:

- Sauté diced carrots, onion, and celery or bok choy in a pot with olive oil until softened.
- Make chicken bone broth by adding chicken bones to cold water and bringing to a boil. Lower the heat and simmer for 1–2 hours.

Strain, then return broth to the pot. (Bone broth can also be purchased at grocery stores for your convenience.)
- Add diced chicken breast, chopped garlic, and chopped herbs such as sage and rosemary.
- Do not overcook—the chicken will get tough. It cooks fully in about 15 minutes.
- Serve hot.

Spicy Lentil Soup:

- Sauté diced carrots, onion, and celery in a pot with olive oil until tender.
- Add dried lentils, chicken bone broth or vegetable broth, diced tomatoes, chopped garlic, and spices such as cumin, oregano, and cayenne pepper.
- Bring to a boil, lower the heat, and simmer until the lentils are tender, about 30–40 minutes.
- Serve hot.

Baked Sweet Potato with Spicy Yogurt Sauce:

- Preheat the oven to 400°F.
- Make several holes in the sweet potato with a fork, then bake until soft.
- In a bowl, mix plain yogurt with chopped garlic, chopped herbs such as cilantro or parsley, and spices such as cumin and cayenne pepper.
- Slice the sweet potato in half and add spicy yogurt sauce on top.

Roasted Brussels Sprouts with Spices:

- Preheat the oven to 400°F.
- Slice Brussels sprouts and coat with olive oil, salt, and pepper.
- Roast until they are tender and crispy, about 30 minutes.
- Mix spicy brown mustard with honey, lemon juice, and herbs such as thyme or rosemary.
- Serve the roasted Brussels sprouts with spicy mustard sauce.

Snacks

1. Warm apple slices with a sprinkle of cinnamon and honey
2. A cup of hot bone broth with ginger and turmeric
3. Sliced cucumber with hummus or guacamole
4. A small bowl of warm oatmeal with sliced banana and walnuts
5. A smoothie with spinach, frozen berries, non-dairy milk, and a portion of protein powder
6. Almonds or other nuts with a piece of fruit
7. A rice cake with avocado and smoked salmon
8. Roasted sweet potato slices with sea salt and olive oil
9. A warm cup of herbal tea with lemon and honey
10. Carrots and celery sticks with almond butter or tahini dip

Foods and Snacks to Avoid

Avoiding certain foods and snacks during the first stage of a cold or flu can help prevent compromising or weakening your immune system and promote faster recovery. Some foods to avoid include:

- Sugary food/snacks compromise the immune system, making it harder for the body to fight off the virus.
- Dairy products can thicken mucus and make congestion worse.
- Fried foods are difficult to digest and contribute to inflammation in the body, which can make it harder for the immune system to knock out a virus.
- Both caffeine and alcohol can dehydrate the body, which can impair immune function and prolong recovery time.
- Spicy foods may irritate the throat and worsen symptoms such as coughing and sore throat.

Support your body with good eating practices. Eat whole foods that are nutritious—such as vegetables and fruits, whole grains, healthy fats, tofu, tempeh, and clean lean protein—to support the immune system and promote faster recovery. Drink plenty of water as well to keep the body hydrated and to help flush out toxins.

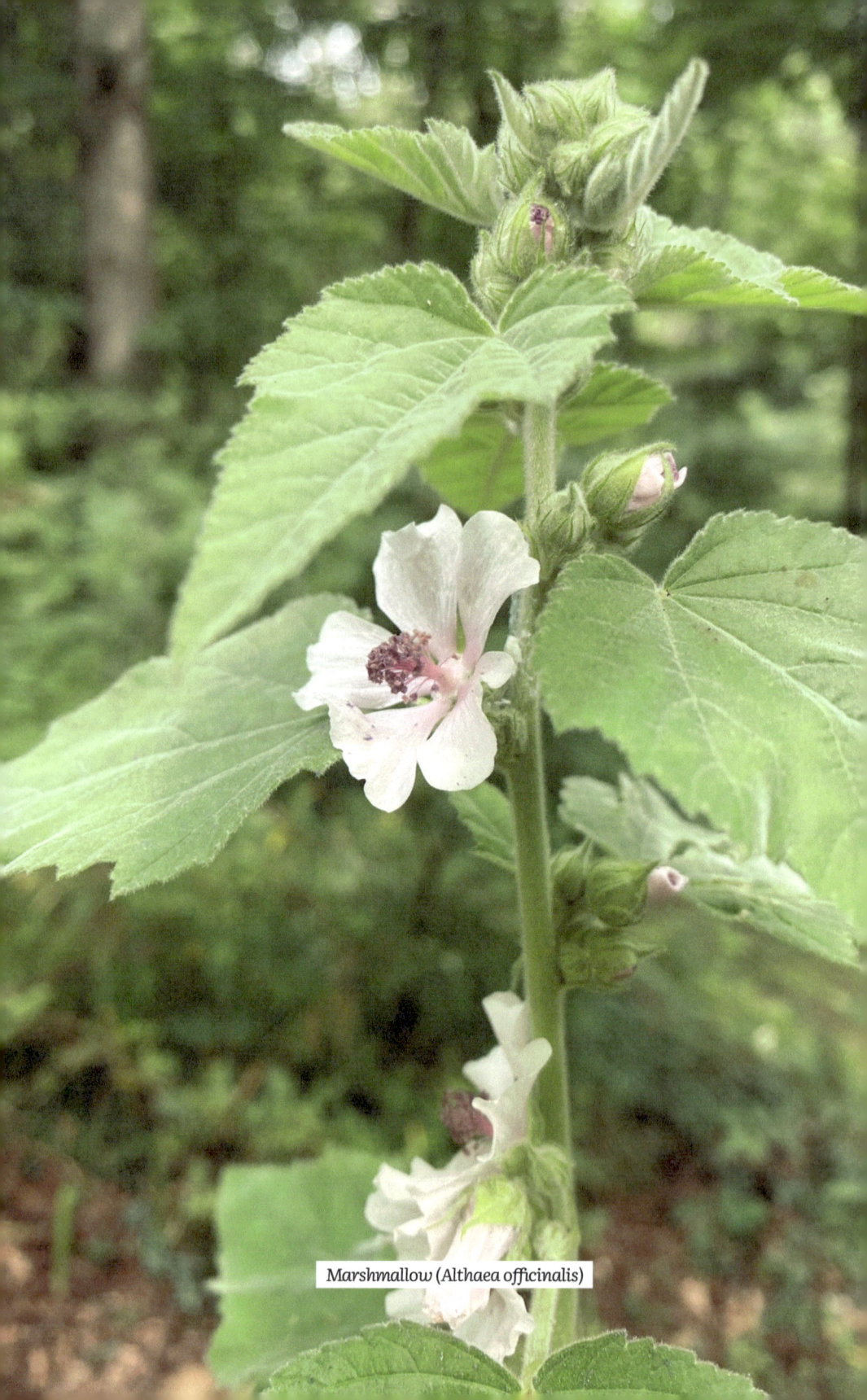

Marshmallow (Althaea officinalis)

CHAPTER 2.
DEMULCENT HERBS

Demulcents are herbs that contain a concentration of mucilaginous substances that adhere to the lining of the tissue. Mucilage is soothing and sticky, making it a great host for stronger, more powerful herbs to stick to tissue, which then helps the body resist the organism. The mucilage creates a wall of protection that prevents inflammatory responses. Mucilage herbs are also hydrating, supporting the flow of the matrix system that the immune system's T and B cells traverse to reach the infected area. These cells are the body's powerful defense for fighting an infection. Mucilage assists the immune system while protecting the body's tissue and organs from inflammation that can make the tissue raw, resulting in a more severe infection and possible bleeding in the organs.

A) Marshmallow (Althaea officinalis)
B) Licorice (Glycyrrhiza glabra)
C) Slippery Elm (Ulmus rubra)
D) Mullein (Verbascum thapsus)
E) Chickweed (Stellaria media)
F) Chamomile (Matricaria chamomilla)

Preparation & Dosage

Marshmallow (Althaea officinalis)

Marshmallow contains a high amount of mucilage. When mixed with water, it forms a thick, soothing coating for irritated tissues. This property makes marshmallow an excellent demulcent herb, as it can soothe and protect the mucous membranes in the body, including the digestive and respiratory systems. This can help relieve coughs, sore throats, and gastrointestinal irritation. Additionally, marshmallow has mild anti-inflammatory and immune-boosting effects, further supporting its use as a demulcent herb.

Marshmallow Leaf Tea Recipe:

When consumed as tea, the mucilage in marshmallow coats the throat, stomach, and intestines, creating a soothing, protective layer that can reduce inflammation and promote healing.

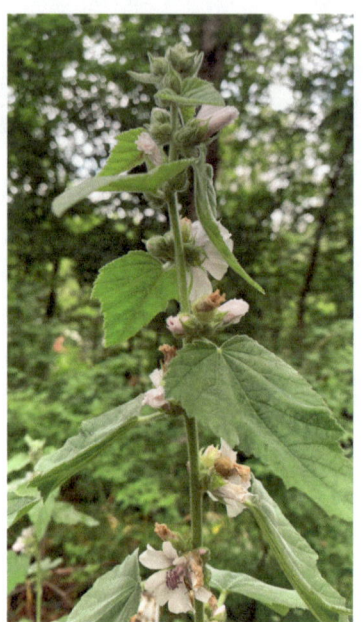

- Place 6 teaspoons of fresh marshmallow leaves OR 3 teaspoons of dried marshmallow leaves into a diffuser.
- Place into a mug and pour simmering water over the marshmallow.
- Steep for 5–7 minutes.
- Sweeten with honey or maple syrup and lemon if desired.
- Drink the tea while it is still warm.

Marshmallow Root Infusion Recipe:

- Bring 2 cups of water to a boil in a pot.
- Place a handful of fresh marshmallow root OR dried marshmallow root into the boiling water.
- Lower to a simmer and cover the pot.
- Simmer to 5–7 minutes.
- Remove from heat and strain the mixture.
- Drink about an ounce of warm tea at a time throughout the day.

Note: Marshmallow tea is safe for most people, but it may be contraindicated with certain medications, such as diabetes drugs. Marshmallow root/leaf may also cause side effects such as stomach aches and allergic reactions in some individuals. As with any herbal remedy, it is best to slowly increase the amount used over time and monitor your body's response. Always consult with a clinical herbalist or a health care professional before taking herbal remedies if you have any concerns.

Licorice (Glycyrrhiza glabra)

Licorice is a demulcent herb that contains glycyrrhizin, a substance that has anti-inflammatory and immune-modulating effects on the body. Its demulcent properties make it effective in soothing and coating irritated mucous membranes, including those in the respiratory and digestive systems.

Licorice has been used traditionally to treat respiratory illnesses such as coughs, colds, bronchitis, and sore throats, and it has also been used to soothe digestive complaints such as heartburn, ulcers, and gastritis. Licorice has been shown to have antiviral properties as well and is regularly used in TCM as an herbal remedy for viral infections such as influenza, hepatitis, and herpes.

Licorice Infusion Recipe:

- Bring 2 cups of water to a boil in a pot.
- Place 2 teaspoons of fresh or dried licorice root into the boiling water.
- Lower to a simmer and cover the pot.
- Simmer for 5–7 minutes.
- Remove from heat.
- Let it steep for 3–5 minutes.
- Strain the mixture and drink one cup at a time. Drink 1–2 cups a day as needed. This tea is meant to be sipped on slowly, an ounce at a time.
- Licorice is naturally sweet; taste before adding natural sweeteners.
- Drink the tea while it is still warm.

Note: Licorice can increase blood pressure and should not be consumed by people with high blood pressure or heart disease. Licorice may also be contraindicated with certain medications, blood thinners and diuretics. As with any herbal remedy, it is best to slowly increase the amount used over time and monitor your body's response. Always consult with a clinical herbalist or a health care professional before taking herbal remedies if you have any concerns.

Slippery Elm (Ulmus rubra)

Slippery elm's inner bark has been traditionally used as an herbal remedy and nutritional purposes for its demulcent and mucilaginous properties. It contains a lot of mucilage and infuses into a slimy carbohydrate that can soothe and protect irritated mucous membranes in the throat, stomach, and intestines.

It has been used for treating sore throat, cough, and gastrointestinal issues like colitis, ulcers, and diarrhea. In addition, it is an anti-inflammatory that can help bring down swelling and irritation in the body. Slippery elm can be consumed as a powder or in capsules, lozenges, and tea. In some countries, slippery elm is eaten as breakfast cereal.

Slippery Elm Infusion Recipe:

- Put 1 teaspoon of slippery elm powder in a mug.
- Pour 1 cup of boiling water over the powder.
- Stir the mixture until it reaches a thick and slimy consistency.
- Add more water or juice if desired.
- Allow the tea to cool slightly before drinking.
- Drink 1–2 cups a day as needed. Drink small amounts throughout the day for better absorption.

Note: Slippery elm may be contraindicated with some medications, including blood thinners and medication for diabetics. Always consult with a clinical herbalist or a health care professional before taking herbal remedies if you have any concerns.

Mullein (Verbascum thapsus)

As it contains a lot of mucilage, mullein is ideal for soothing sore throats, dry coughs, and irritated lungs. In addition to its demulcent properties, mullein has many herbal actions:

1. Mullein is an expectorant. It may loosen mucus from the respiratory tract, making it a useful remedy for coughs and lung congestion.
2. Mullein has anti-inflammatory compounds, making it useful for reducing inflammation in the respiratory tract and other parts of the body.
3. Mullein has analgesic actions. It has mild pain-relieving properties, making it useful for soothing sore throats and other painful conditions.
4. Mullein's antimicrobial properties can help to fight off infections in the respiratory tract.

Mullein Infusion Recipe:

- Combine 1 tablespoon total of mullein leaves and flowers in an infuser and place it in a mug.
- Pour 1 cup of simmering water onto the herbs.
- Steep for 5–7 minutes.
- Sweeten with honey or maple syrup if desired.
- Drink the tea while it is still warm.
- Drink 1–2 cups per day, sipping slowly throughout the day.

Mullein Tincture Recipe:

- Put dried mullein leaves and/or flowers into a jar.
- Pour in enough alcohol to cover, leaving space at the top.*

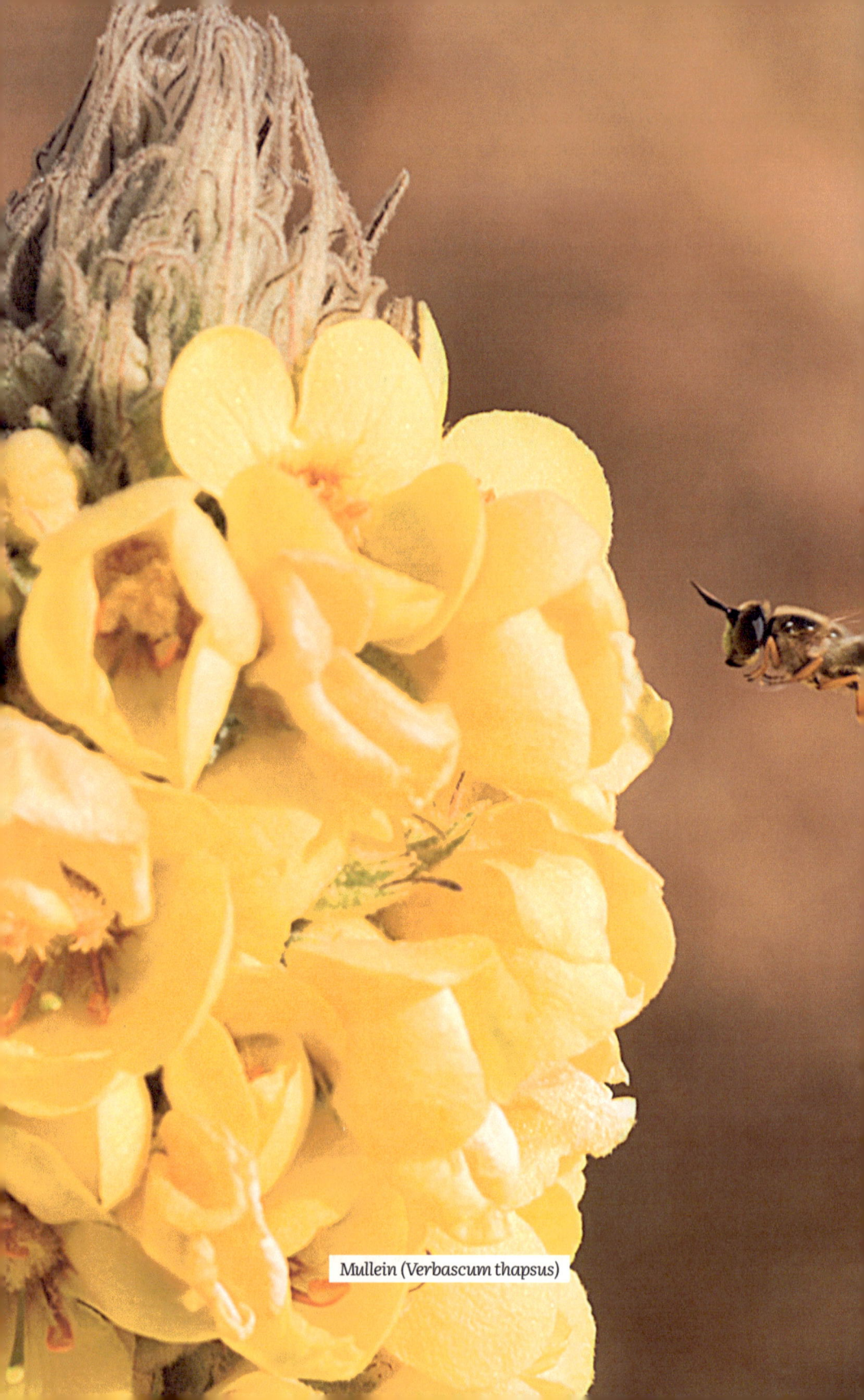
Mullein (Verbascum thapsus)

- Tightly seal the jar, label, date, and shake well.
- Let it steep for 2–3 months. Shake the jar weekly.
- Strain the mixture, then store it in a glass jar in a dark place.
- Take 10–15 drops diluted in a little bit of water up to three times a day as needed.
- For children, the proper amount will vary depending on their age and weight. Use 3–5 drops diluted in a small amount of juice or water up to three times a day as needed.

Mullein Capsules:

- Mullein capsules are available commercially and should be taken according to the directions on the label.

Note: Mullein is contraindicated with certain medications such as blood thinners and diabetes medications. As with any herbal remedy, it is best to slowly increase the amount used over time and monitor your body's response. Always consult with a clinical herbalist or a health care professional before taking herbal remedies if you have any concerns.

Chickweed (Stellaria media)

Chickweed is an herb that has multiple synergistic actions for the lungs and kidneys when fighting a cold, flu, and other viruses. It is an expectorant, demulcent, and a diuretic. As a demulcent with a high mucilage content, chickweed is used to coat, soothe, and protect irritated mucous membranes.

Chickweed Infusion Recipe:

- Put 1 heaping tablespoon of fresh chickweed OR 2 teaspoons of dried chickweed into a infuser.
- Place into a mug and pour simmering water over the herbs.
- Steep for 5–7 minutes.

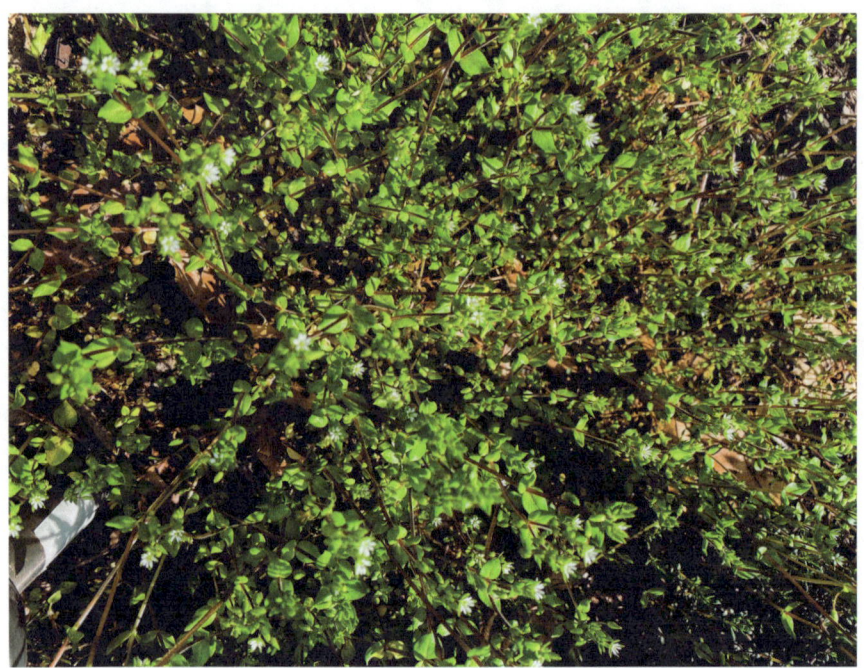

- Sweeten with honey or maple syrup and lemon if desired.
- Drink the tea while it is still warm.
- Drink 1–2 cups per day, sipping slowly throughout the day.

Chickweed Tincture Recipe:

- Wash and chop fresh chickweed and place it in a jar.
- Pour in enough alcohol to cover, leaving space at the top.*
- Tightly seal the jar, label, date, and shake well.
- Let it steep for 2–3 months. Shake the jar weekly.
- Strain the mixture, then store it in a glass jar in a dark place.
- Take 10–15 drops diluted in a little bit of water up to three times a day as needed.
- For children, the proper amount will vary depending on their age and weight. Use 5–7 drops diluted in a small amount of juice or water up to three times a day as needed.

Note: Chickweed may be contraindicated with certain medications such as blood thinners and diabetes medications. As with any herbal remedy, it is best to slowly increase the amount used over time and monitor your body's response. Always consult with a clinical herbalist or a health care professional before taking herbal remedies if you have any concerns.

Chamomile (Matricaria chamomilla)

Chamomile is a demulcent used for soothing irritated internal tissues. Chamomile prepared as tea will settle bloating, cramping, indigestion, and digestive spasms. It also speeds up the healing process of mucous membranes in the colon and stomach.

Chamomile Infusion Recipe:

- Put 1 tablespoon of dried chamomile flowers in an infuser.
- Pour a cup of simmering water onto the chamomile.
- Steep for 5-7 minutes.
- Drink 1–3 mugs a day as needed.

Chamomile Tincture Recipe:

- Fill a clean jar with dried chamomile flowers.
- Pour in enough alcohol to cover, leaving space at the top.*
- Tightly seal the jar, label, date, and shake well.
- Let it steep for 2–3 months. Shake the jar weekly.
- Strain the mixture, then store it in a glass jar in a dark place.
- Take 15–20 drops diluted in a small amount of water up to three times a day as needed.
- For children, the proper amount will vary depending on their age and weight. Use 3–7 drops diluted in a small amount of juice or water up to three times a day as needed.

Note: Always consult with a clinical herbalist or a health care professional before taking herbal remedies if you have any concerns.

Demulcent Food & Dosage

This first recipe makes a delicious and nutritious breakfast or snack!

Carob is considered a demulcent herb with anti-inflammatory and antioxidant properties. Its mucilaginous properties help coat and protect the mucous membranes of the digestive system and the respiratory system. It is also considered an expectorant, helping to loosen and expel mucus from the respiratory system.

Oatmeal provides fiber and complex carbohydrates for sustained energy, while almond or coconut yogurt each offer protein and probiotics for gut health. The unsweetened carob chips can add a touch of sweetness and provide demulcent properties to help soothe the digestive tract. The berries are demulcent as well and loaded with vitamins and minerals.

Oatmeal, Unsweetened Non-Dairy Yogurt, and **Unsweetened Carob Chips:**

Ingredients:

- ½ cup raw or cooked rolled oats (or any other rolled whole grain used as a cereal)
- 1 cup unsweetened non-dairy yogurt
- 1 tablespoon unsweetened carob chips
- Berries for topping

Instructions:

- Put rolled whole grains into a bowl.
- Cook the rolled oats according to package directions.
- Top the oats with unsweetened yogurt.
- Sprinkle the unsweetened carob chips on top.
- Add berries.
- Enjoy your delicious and nourishing breakfast or snack!

Unsweetened Carob Chip Cookie Recipe:

Ingredients:

- 1 cup almond or stone-ground whole wheat flour
- ¼ cup coconut or whole grain flour
- ½ tsp baking soda
- ¼ tsp salt
- ¼ cup melted virgin coconut oil
- ¼ cup natural sweetener (honey or maple syrup)
- 1 egg
- 1 tsp vanilla extract
- ½ cup unsweetened carob chips

Instructions:

- Preheat oven to 350°F.
- Line a baking sheet with parchment paper.
- In a bowl, add almond flour, coconut, or whole grain flour, baking soda, and salt and whisk together.
- In a separate bowl, whisk together the coconut oil, honey or maple syrup, egg, and vanilla extract.
- Pour the wet ingredients into the dry ingredients ⅓ at a time and stir until well combined.
- Fold in unsweetened carob chips.
- Scoop the dough onto the baking sheet with a melon scooper. Space the cookies about 2 inches apart.
- Bake for 12–15 minutes until the edges are golden brown.
- Allow the cookies to cool on the baking sheet before transferring them onto a wire rack to completely cool.

Enjoy these demulcent carob chip cookies as a soothing treat!

Carob Candy:

Ingredients:

- 1 cup unsweetened carob chips
- ½ cup natural sweetener (honey or maple syrup)
- ½ cup virgin coconut oil
- 1 tsp vanilla extract
- ½ tsp sea salt

Instructions:

- In a double boiler, melt the carob chips and virgin coconut oil together.
- Remove from heat, then stir in the natural sweetener, vanilla extract, and sea salt.
- Drizzle the mixture into a candy mold or onto a baking sheet lined with parchment paper.
- Place in the fridge or freezer until set.
- Pop the candy out of molds while still cold.
- Eat as a treat or melt into warm milk or water for a soothing demulcent beverage.

Note: Staying hydrated is important when you have a cold, flu, or any other virus. Proper water intake helps to prevent dehydration, thin mucus, and reduce congestion.

Hydrating Snack and Drink Recipes:

- Citrus Water: Slice some oranges, lemons, and limes and add them to a pitcher of water. Let it cool and infuse in the fridge for a few hours to flavor the citrus water. Drink throughout the day.
- Herbal Tea: Brew some herbal tea, such as chamomile, peppermint, or ginger tea. These teas can help soothe sore throat and ease nausea.

- Coconut Water: Drink coconut water to replenish your body with essential minerals. It is a great natural source of electrolytes, which are important for hydration.
- Smoothies: Make a fruit smoothie with ingredients like bananas, strawberries, and blueberries. Add some spinach or kale for added vitamins and minerals.
- Broth: Sip on warm bone or vegetable broth throughout the day. The warm liquid can help soothe a sore throat, and the added electrolytes can help prevent dehydration.

It is also important to avoid drinks that can dehydrate you, such as alcohol, coffee, and sugary drinks. These can worsen dehydration and make your symptoms worse.

Hydrating Snacks

- Water-rich fruits such as watermelon, cantaloupe, oranges, grapefruit, and berries.
- Vegetables with high water content such as cucumbers, celery, lettuce, spinach, and zucchini.
- Broth-based soups such as chicken soup, miso soup, or vegetable broth.
- Smoothies made with water or coconut water, fresh or frozen fruit, and leafy greens.
- Herbal teas such as peppermint, ginger, chamomile, or echinacea tea.
- Electrolyte-rich beverages such as coconut water or sports drinks (in moderation).
- Snacks such as watermelon slices, cucumber sticks, celery and carrot sticks, or a fresh fruit salad with a drizzle of honey or maple syrup.

It is important to stay hydrated during illness to help flush out toxins, keep mucus membranes moist, and support the immune system.

Foods and Substances to Avoid When Using Demulcents

- Spicy and acidic foods, tomatoes, citrus fruits, and vinegar can irritate the throat and exacerbate the symptoms of a sore throat.
- Dairy products such as milk can increase mucus production and worsen congestion.
- Alcohol and caffeine can be dehydrating and irritating to the throat and stomach.
- Fried and fatty foods are difficult to digest and can irritate the stomach.
- Sugary food and processed foods can weaken the immune system and worsen inflammation.

It is important to stick to a whole foods diet when using demulcents to support the body's health and healing process.

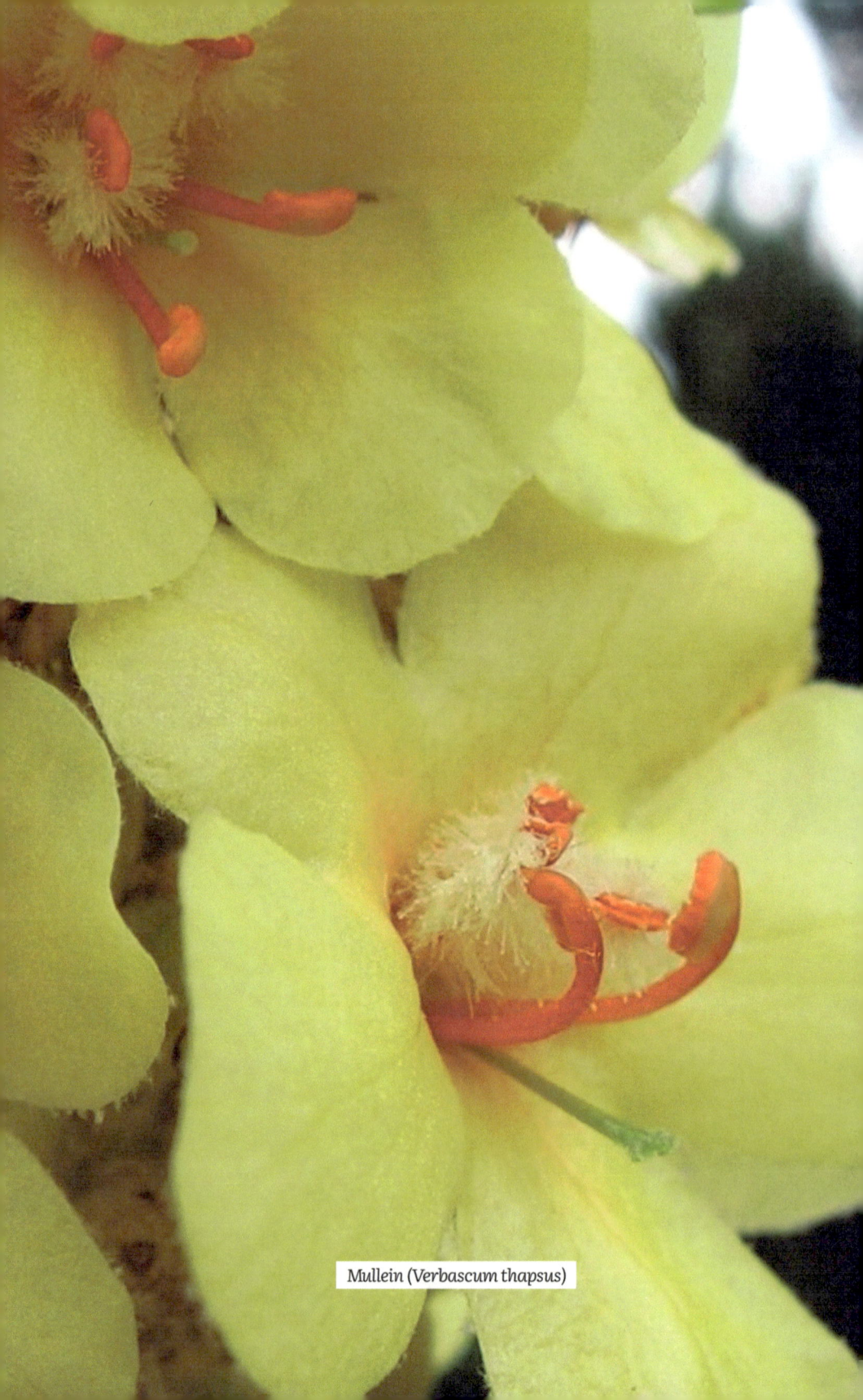
Mullein (Verbascum thapsus)

CHAPTER 3.
EXPECTORANT HERBS

It is important to keep stress levels low when fighting a virus. Stress can weaken the immune system, making it much more difficult for the body to fight off viruses and viral infections. When the immune system is compromised, this can lead to an increase in mucus production and respiratory symptoms. However, stress itself does not directly

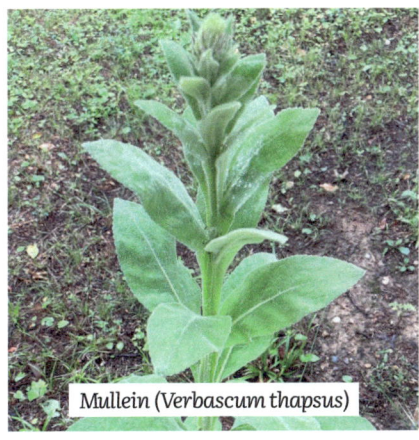
Mullein (Verbascum thapsus)

create more mucus; it is the body's stress response while fighting the infection that results in increased mucus production. Therefore, it is important to manage stress levels during an illness—less stress means less impact on the mucus system and more support for the immune system's ability to fight infections.

An expectorant helps to loosen and expel mucus from the respiratory tract, making it easier to cough up mucus and clear the airways. Expectorants stimulate the production and secretion of thinner, less viscous mucus in the airways that can then be coughed up more easily.

Some expectorants work by directly affecting the viscosity of mucus, making it thinner and easier to move. These include marshmallow, licorice, elecampane, thyme, and mullein. Other expectorants work to free the lungs by irritating the respiratory tract and stimulating an increase of mucus production and coughing. Eucalyptus and menthol work this way.

Many natural expectorants, such as thyme, mullein, and licorice, contain compounds that have mucolytic (mucus-breaking) and expectorant properties. For example, thyme contains thymol and carvacrol, which are known to thin mucus and increase coughing, while mullein contains mucilage, which soothes irritated airways and helps to expel mucus.

A) Mullein (Verbascum thapsus)
B) Thyme (Thymus vulgaris)
C) Licorice (Glycyrrhiza glabra)
D) Elecampane (Inula helenium)
E) Coltsfoot (Tussilago farfara)
F) Chickweed (Stellaria media)
G) Marshmallow (Althaea officinalis)
H) Hyssop (Hyssopus officinalis)

A Note About Herbal Expectorants:

Preparation methods for expectorant herbs can include teas, syrups, inhalations, and steam baths. It is important to use caution with expectorants, as excessive use can lead to dehydration and electrolyte imbalances. It is recommended to increase your fluids and rest properly when using expectorants to support the immune system during a viral infection.

Preparation & Dosage

Mullein (Verbascum thapsus)

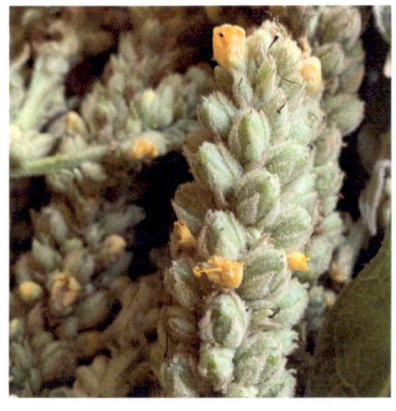

Mullein is an herb commonly used to help clear the respiratory tract of mucus and phlegm. Mullein may promote the healthy function of the respiratory system and improve breathing, as it contains compounds called saponins that can help break up mucus and make it easier to cough up. Mullein also has anti-inflammatory properties that can help soothe the respiratory tract, making it less irritated and inflamed. Additionally, mullein is a mild analgesic, which means it may help alleviate pain associated with coughing.

Mullein Infusion Recipe:

- Add 4 teaspoons of fresh mullein leaves OR 2 teaspoons of dried leaves to an infuser.
- Place into a mug and pour simmering water over the herbs.
- Steep for 5–7 minutes.
- Add honey and lemon if desired.
- For a stronger tea, you can use more mullein.

Mullein Tincture Recipe:

- Cut fresh mullein leaves and flowers into small pieces and place in a jar.
- Pour in enough alcohol to cover, leaving space at the top.*
- Tightly seal the jar, label, date, and shake well.
- Let it steep for 2–3 months. Shake the jar weekly.
- Strain the mixture, then store it in a glass jar in a dark place.
- Take 10–20 drops diluted into a little bit of water, up to three times a day.
- For children, the proper amount will vary depending on their age and weight. Use 3–5 drops diluted in a small amount of juice or water up to three times a day as needed.

Mullein Syrup Expectorant:

Ingredients:

- 1 cup dried mullein leaves OR 2 cups of fresh mullein leaves and flowers
- 4 cups water
- 2 cups honey or agave syrup
- Fresh juice of 1 lemon

Instructions:

- Combine the mullein leaves and water in a large pot. Simmer for about 30 minutes, or until the liquid has evaporated to about half the amount.
- Strain the mixture through cheesecloth, then squeeze the herbs to extract as much liquid as possible.
- Pour the liquid back into the pot and add the natural sweetener (honey or maple syrup) and lemon juice. Stir well.
- Heat the mixture again on low heat. Stir occasionally until the syrup has thickened.
- Remove from heat and let cool.
- Transfer the syrup to a bottle. Store it in the refrigerator for up to three months.
- Take 1–2 tablespoons up to three times per day as needed.
- For children, the proper amount will vary depending on their age and weight. Use 1–2 teaspoons up to three times a day as needed.

Note: Mullein may cause allergic reactions in some individuals. The safety of long-term or high-dose use is not currently well-established. As with any herbal remedy, it is best to slowly increase the amount used over time and monitor your body's response. Always consult with a clinical herbalist or health care professional before taking herbal remedies, particularly if you have a health-related condition or are taking medication.

Thyme (Thymus vulgaris)

A natural expectorant that helps to fight respiratory infections, thyme aids in loosening and expelling mucus from the lungs and respiratory tract. It contains compounds that can break down and thin out mucus, making it easier to cough up. It also serves as an antiseptic that cleanses mucus from the lungs, soothes coughs, and fights nasal congestion.

Thyme is often used as a remedy to relieve symptoms of viral infections such as coughs, congestion, and sore throats. However, it is important to note that while thyme may have some antiviral properties, it should not be used as a single herb for viral infections but added for its virtue as an expectorant.

Thyme Infusion Recipe:

- Cut a handful of fresh thyme OR use 2–3 teaspoons of dried thyme and place it into a tea ball or tea bag.
- Place into a cup and pour simmering water over the herbs.
- Steep for 5–7 minutes.
- Add honey or maple syrup if desired.
- For a stronger tea, use more thyme.

Thyme Tincture Recipe:

- Cut fresh thyme leaves into small pieces and place in a jar.
- Pour in enough alcohol to cover, leaving space at the top.*
- Tightly seal the jar, label, date, and shake well.
- Let it steep for 2–3 months. Shake the jar weekly.
- Take 3–5 drops diluted in an ounce of water or juice twice a day (once in the morning and once in evening).
- For children, the proper amount will vary depending on their age and weight. Use 2–3 drops diluted in a small amount of water or juice up to three times a day as needed.

Note: Thyme may interact with certain medications and may cause side effects such as stomachaches or allergic reactions in some individuals. As with any herbal remedy, it is best to slowly increase the amount used over time and monitor your body's response. Always consult with a clinical herbalist or health care professional before taking herbal remedies, particularly if you have a health-related condition or are taking medication.

Licorice (Glycyrrhiza glabra)

Licorice has several effects on the body, including expectorant, anti-inflammatory, demulcent, and adrenal tonic actions.

As an expectorant, licorice works by stimulating the production of mucus in the respiratory tract. This increased mucus production helps to moisten and soothe irritated or inflamed respiratory tissues, making it easier to cough up phlegm and other respiratory secretions. Licorice also contains compounds that have antiviral and antibacterial properties that help support the immune system in fighting off respiratory infections.

Licorice also has a demulcent action, meaning that it forms a soothing protective layer over irritated or inflamed mucous membranes in the respiratory, digestive, and urinary systems. This can help to relieve symptoms such as sore throat, cough, and indigestion.

Finally, licorice has an adrenal tonic action, which means that it helps to support and strengthen the adrenal glands responsible for producing hormones that regulate the body's stress response. This can help to improve energy levels and reduce stress and anxiety.

Licorice Infusion Recipe:

- Add 2–4 teaspoons of fresh licorice root OR 1–2 teaspoons of chopped/crushed pieces of dried licorice to a pot with 2 cups of water.
- Bring to a simmer and let the herbs simmer for 5 minutes.
- Remove from heat.
- Steep for 5–10 minutes, then strain.

- Add lemon or aromatic herbs for flavor if desired.
- For a stronger tea, you can use more licorice root.
- Drink 1–3 cups of licorice tea a day as needed.

Licorice Tincture Recipe:

- Chop fresh or dried licorice root into small pieces and place in a jar.
- Pour in enough alcohol to cover, leaving space at the top.*
- Tightly seal the jar, label, date, and shake well.
- Let it steep for 2–3 months. Shake the jar weekly.
- Strain and store it in a glass jar.
- Take 10–15 drops diluted in a little bit of water up to three times a day as needed.
- For children, the proper amount will vary depending on their age and weight. Use 3–5 drops diluted in a small amount of water or juice up to three times a day as needed.

Note: Licorice should be used with caution by individuals with high blood pressure. Licorice may also interact with certain medications and can cause allergic reactions in some individuals. As with any herbal remedy, it is best to slowly increase the amount used over time and monitor your body's response. Always consult with a clinical herbalist or health care professional before taking herbal remedies, particularly if you have a health-related condition or are taking medication.

Elecampane (Inula helenium)

Elecampane contains inulin and other mucilage compounds that help to soothe and moisten the respiratory tract, making it easier to cough up and expel mucus. It also contains volatile oils such as camphene and pinene that possess expectorant properties to help loosen and thin mucus in the lungs and nasal passages. Elecampane's antibacterial properties can also help to fight off respiratory infections and reduce inflammation in the respiratory system. These properties make elecampane an effective expectorant for treating coughs, bronchitis, and other respiratory conditions.

Elecampane Infusion Recipe:

- Add 2–4 teaspoons of fresh elecampane root OR c2 teaspoons of dried elecampane root to a pot with 2 cups of water.
- Bring to a simmer and allow the herbs to simmer for 10–15 minutes.
- Remove from heat, then strain.
- Add honey or maple syrup for sweetness if desired.
- For a stronger tea, use more elecampane root.
- Drink up to three cups per day as needed.

Elecampane Tincture Recipe:

- Chop fresh elecampane root into pieces and place in a jar.
- Pour in enough alcohol to cover, leaving space at the top.*
- Tightly seal the jar, label, date, and shake well.
- Let it steep for 2–3 months. Shake the jar weekly.
- Strain and store it in a glass jar.
- Take 10–20 drops diluted in a little bit of juice or water up to three times a day as needed.
- For children, the proper amount will vary depending on their age and weight. Use 3–5 drops diluted in a small amount of water or juice up to three times a day as needed.

Note: Elecampane should be used with caution by individuals with allergies to other plants in the Asteraceae family, as it may cause allergic reactions. Elecampane may be contraindicated with certain medications and should not be used by individuals with a history of seizures. As with any herbal remedy, it is best to slowly increase the amount used over time and monitor your body's response. Always consult with a clinical herbalist or health care professional before taking herbal remedies, particularly if you have a health-related condition or are taking medication.

Coltsfoot (Tussilago farfara)

Coltsfoot has been used throughout history as an herbal remedy for respiratory conditions. It is a powerful expectorant that helps to loosen and expel mucus from the lungs. Coltsfoot contains mucilage, a sticky substance that can soothe irritated tissues in the respiratory tract, and this makes it effective in reducing inflammation and helping to clear congestion.

Coltsfoot is also a natural cough suppressant, making it beneficial for those with persistent coughs. It works by relaxing the muscles in the bronchial tubes, which can help to reduce coughing fits.

In addition to mucilage, coltsfoot also contains saponins that can break up mucus and loosen and expel phlegm from the respiratory tract.

Coltsfoot has a soothing effect on irritated mucous membranes, helping to reduce inflammation, swelling, and irritation in the respiratory tract.

As an antitussive, coltsfoot can help to reduce coughing, both by soothing irritated tissues and by reducing the sensitivity of the cough reflex.

Coltsfoot also has antimicrobial properties, meaning it may help to fight off infections in the respiratory tract.

Overall, coltsfoot is a helpful herb for conditions affecting the respiratory tract such as coughs, bronchitis, and asthma. However, it is important to note that coltsfoot contains pyrrolizidine alkaloids, which can be toxic in large amounts or with long-term use. As such, it should only be used under the guidance of a clinical herbalist or a qualified healthcare professional.

Coltsfoot Infusion Recipe:

- Put 3–4 teaspoons of fresh coltsfoot leaves OR 2 teaspoons of dried coltsfoot leaves in a mug.
- Pour simmering water over the herbs.
- Steep for 5–7 minutes.
- Strain and drink.
- Add honey or maple syrup if desired.
- For a stronger tea, you can use more coltsfoot leaves.
- Drink up to 3 cups of coltsfoot tea per day as needed.

Coltsfoot Tincture Recipe:

- Chop fresh or dried coltsfoot leaves into small pieces and place in a jar.
- Pour in enough alcohol to cover, leaving space at the top.*
- Tightly seal the jar, label, date, and shake well.
- Let it steep for 2–3 months. Shake the jar weekly.
- Strain and store the tincture in a glass jar.
- Take 10–20 drops diluted in a little bit of juice or water up to three times a day as needed.
- For children, the proper amount will vary depending on their age and weight. Use 3–5 drops diluted in a small amount of juice or water up to three times a day as needed.

Note: Coltsfoot should not be used for prolonged periods of time, as it contains compounds that may be toxic to the liver. Coltsfoot should also be avoided by individuals with a history of liver disease or alcoholism and should be avoided by pregnant or breastfeeding women. As with any herbal remedy, it is best to slowly increase the amount used over time and monitor your body's response. Always consult with a clinical herbalist or health care professional before taking herbal remedies, particularly if you have a health-related condition or are taking medication.

Chickweed (Stellaria media)

Chickweed can soothe inflamed mucus membranes and expel mucus secretions from the lungs, helping to clear and ease congestion. Chickweed contains saponins, compounds that help to break down mucus and make it easier to expel from the respiratory system. This makes chickweed an effective expectorant that can help to relieve coughs and congestion associated with respiratory infections such as the common cold, flu, and other viruses.

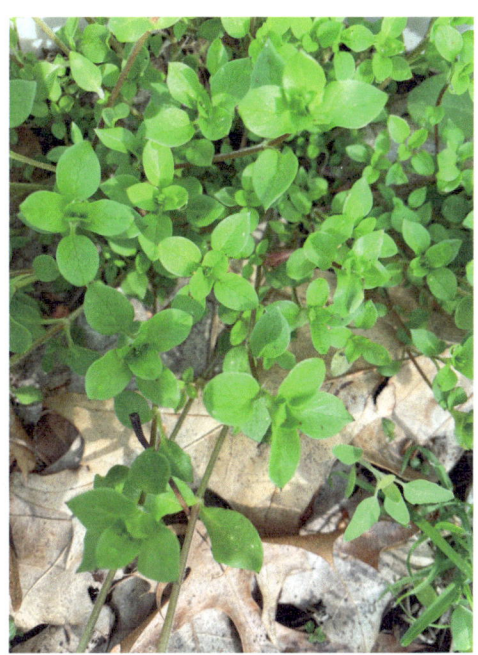

Chickweed Infusion Recipe:

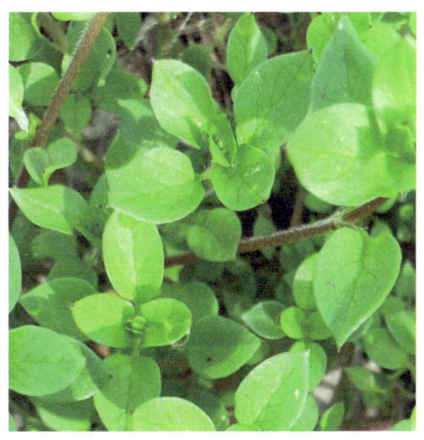

- For fresh chickweed, gather a handful of fresh herbs and add to a mug.
- Pour simmering water over the herbs.
- Steep for 3–5 minutes, strain, and drink while it is warm.
- If using dried chickweed leaves, add 2–3 tablespoons to a mug.
- Pour simmering water over the herbs.
- Steep for 5 minutes, then strain and drink.
- Add honey, maple syrup, or other aromatic herbs for flavor if desired.

- For a stronger tea, you can use more chickweed.
- Drink 2–3 cups of tea a day as needed.

Chickweed Tincture Recipe:

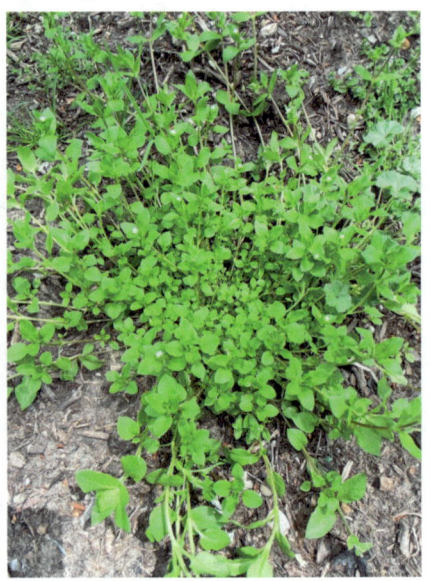

- Rinse and dry off fresh chickweed leaves and flowers thoroughly.
- Chop the herbs finely and put them in a clean glass jar.
- Pour in enough alcohol to cover, leaving space at the top.*
- Tightly seal the jar, label, date, and shake well.
- Let it steep for 2–3 months. Shake the jar weekly.
- Strain the mixture through cheesecloth or fine-mesh strainer, squeezing out as much liquid as possible.
- Transfer the tincture into a clean glass jar and store in a dark place.
- Use 15–20 drops up to three times a day as needed.
- For children, the proper amount will vary depending on their age and weight. Use 5–7 drops diluted in a small amount of juice or water up to three times a day as needed.

Note: Chickweed may cause side effects such as stomachaches and allergic reactions in some individuals. Chickweed may also be contraindicated with certain medications. As with any herbal remedy, it is best to slowly increase the amount used over time and monitor your body's response. Always consult with a clinical herbalist or health care professional before taking herbal remedies, particularly if you have a health-related condition or are taking medication.

Marshmallow (Althaea officinalis)

Marshmallow works as an expectorant by soothing and moistening the mucous membranes in the respiratory tract. Its high mucilage content helps to loosen and thin out mucus, making it less sticky and easier to cough up. Marshmallow also has anti-inflammatory properties that may reduce irritation and inflammation in the respiratory tract, which further supports its expectorant actions.

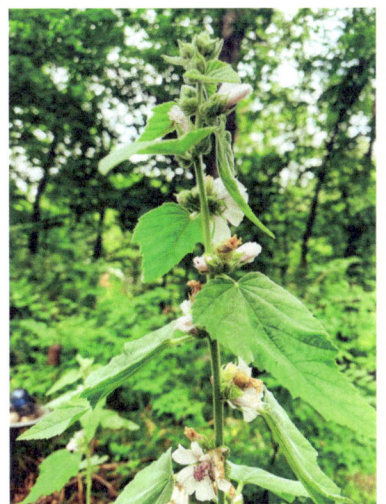

Marshmallow Root Infusion Recipe:

- Place 2–3 teaspoons of dried marshmallow root in a pot with 2 cups of water.
- Bring to a simmer and cover.
- Simmer for 10 minutes.
- Turn off the heat and let the herbs steep for 10 minutes.
- Strain the tea into a mug.
- Add honey or maple syrup and lemon to taste if desired.
- Drink the tea while it is still warm.
- Drink 2–3 cups a day as needed.

Marshmallow Root Tincture Recipe:

- Finely grind the root (either fresh or dried) using a mortar and pestle or blender. Place in a jar.
- Pour in enough alcohol to cover, leaving space at the top.*
- Tightly seal the jar, label, date, and shake well.
- Let it steep for 2–3 months. Shake the jar weekly.
- Strain the mixture and store in a clean jar or bottle.
- Take 15–20 drops diluted in a little bit of water up to three times a day as needed.

- For children, the proper amount will vary depending on their age and weight. Use 5–7 drops diluted in a small amount of juice or water up to three times a day as needed.

Note: Always consult with a clinical herbalist or health care professional before taking herbal remedies, particularly if you have a health-related condition or are taking medication.

Hyssop (Hyssopus officinalis)

Hyssop contains compounds called marrubin and rosmarinic acid that have expectorant properties. These compounds help to loosen and expel mucus from the lungs and respiratory tract by increasing the production of bronchial secretions.

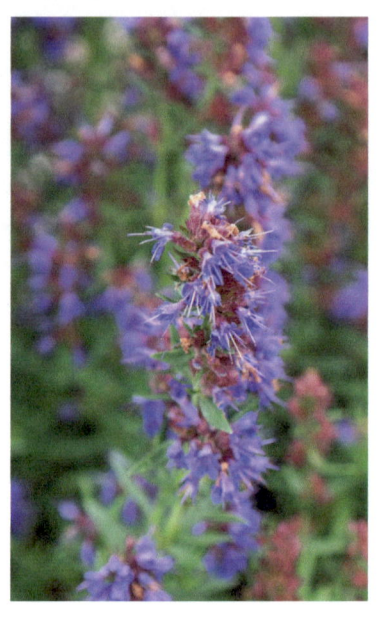

Additionally, hyssop is an effective anti-inflammatory that may reduce inflammation in the respiratory system and promote healing for irritated tissues. Its antiseptic and antiviral properties may also help to fight off infections that can cause congestion and coughing.

Hyssop can be a useful herb for promoting clear lungs and supporting respiratory health. It has a number of other properties and uses as well, including:

- Expectorant: Hyssop can help to loosen and expel mucus from the respiratory tract.
- Antiseptic: Hyssop contains compounds that have antimicrobial properties, making it useful for treating infections.

- Carminative: Hyssop can help to ease digestive discomfort and relieve gas.
- Diaphoretic: Hyssop can help to promote sweating and reduce fevers.
- Nervine: Hyssop promotes a calming effect on the nervous system that may help to reduce anxiety and tension.
- Emmenagogue: Hyssop can stimulate menstrual flow and regulate menstrual cycles.
- Astringent: Hyssop can help to constrict and tighten tissues, making it useful for treating conditions such as diarrhea and hemorrhoids.
- Antispasmodic: Hyssop can help to relieve muscle spasms and cramping.

However, it should be used with caution, as hyssop can be toxic in large doses. It is also not recommended for use during pregnancy or by individuals with epilepsy. Always consult with a clinical herbalist or a qualified health care professional before using any herbal remedy.

Hyssop Infusion Recipe:

- Place 2 tablespoons fresh hyssop leaves OR 1 tablespoon dried hyssop in a tea ball.
- Put the tea ball in a mug and pour simmering water over the leaves.
- Steep for 10 minutes.
- Add honey or maple syrup and lemon if desired
- Enjoy warm and drink 2–3 mugs per day as needed.

Hyssop Tincture Recipe:

- Fill a jar halfway with hyssop leaves and flowers.
- Pour in enough alcohol to cover, leaving space at the top.*
- Tightly seal the jar, label, date, and shake well.
- Let it steep for 2–3 months. Shake the jar weekly.

- Strain the mixture, then store it in a glass jar in a dark place.
- Use 10–20 drops of hyssop tincture up to three times a day.
- For children, the proper amount will vary depending on their age and weight. Use 3–5 drops diluted in a small amount of juice or water up to three times a day as needed.

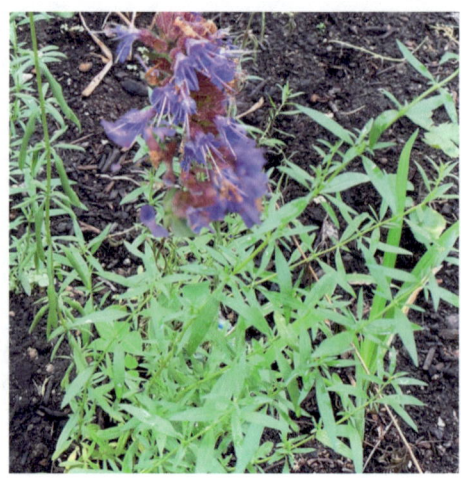

Hyssop Steam Vapor:

- Place ¼ - ½ cup of fresh hyssop leaves and flowers in a large bowl.
- Pour 2 cups of simmering water over the plant material.
- Lean over the bowl, covering your head and the bowl with a towel to trap the steam.
- Breathe deeply and inhale the steam for 10–15 minutes.
- Try hyssop steam inhalation once or twice a day.

Expectorant Food & Recipes

Food and Self-Care for Congestion

- Chicken Soup: The steam from the hot soup can help loosen up mucus, and the nutrients in the chicken can help boost your immune system.
- Spicy Foods: Spicy foods like chili peppers, horseradish, and wasabi can help break up congestion and clear your sinuses. A spicy chili can help loosen up mucus and support the immune system.

- Garlic: Garlic has natural antibacterial properties that can help fight off infections that cause congestion.
- Ginger Tea: Ginger is a natural anti-inflammatory that can help relieve congestion. Try some ginger tea by steeping sliced ginger in simmered water and adding honey and lemon.
- Citrus Fruits: Vitamin C supports the immune system and may help reduce inflammation. Oranges, lemons, and grapefruits are high in vitamin C.
- Steam Inhalation: Inhaling steam can help loosen up mucus and relieve congestion. You can add eucalyptus or peppermint essential oils to the hot water for added relief.
- Saline Nasal Rinse: Nasal rinses help clear out mucus and relieve congestion. To make your own saline solution, combine ¼ teaspoon of finely grated salt with 1 cup of warm water and stir until dissolved.
- Turmeric Milk: Turmeric has natural anti-inflammatory properties that can help relieve congestion. You can make turmeric milk by adding turmeric, honey or maple syrup, and ginger to warm non-dairy milk. If using fresh ginger, let it steep for 5–10 minutes.
- Warm Compress: A warm compress of marshmallow can help relieve congestion by opening the sinuses. You can soak a washcloth in hot marshmallow tea and place it over your face.
- Bone Broth: Any type of bone broth can be beneficial for congestion, but chicken bone broth is often recommended because it has a high concentration of the amino acid cysteine, which may thin mucus and reduce inflammation in the respiratory system. Additionally, adding aromatic herbs such as thyme and oregano can further support respiratory health and enhance the flavor of the broth.

Foods to Avoid When Congested

Avoid the following foods that may contribute to inflammation and mucus production.

- Dairy products increase mucus production.
- Fried foods irritate the mucus lining and contribute to inflammation.
- Processed foods contain ingredients that may worsen congestion and inflammation.
- Sugary foods may also contribute to inflammation and weaken the immune system.

Instead, it is best to focus on whole foods that are nutrient dense, such as fruits, vegetables, whole grains, tofu, tempeh, and lean proteins. These foods are ideal for supporting the immune system and overall health. Additionally, consuming warm fluids like herbal teas, bone broth, and warm coconut milk or water can help to soothe congestion and support hydration.

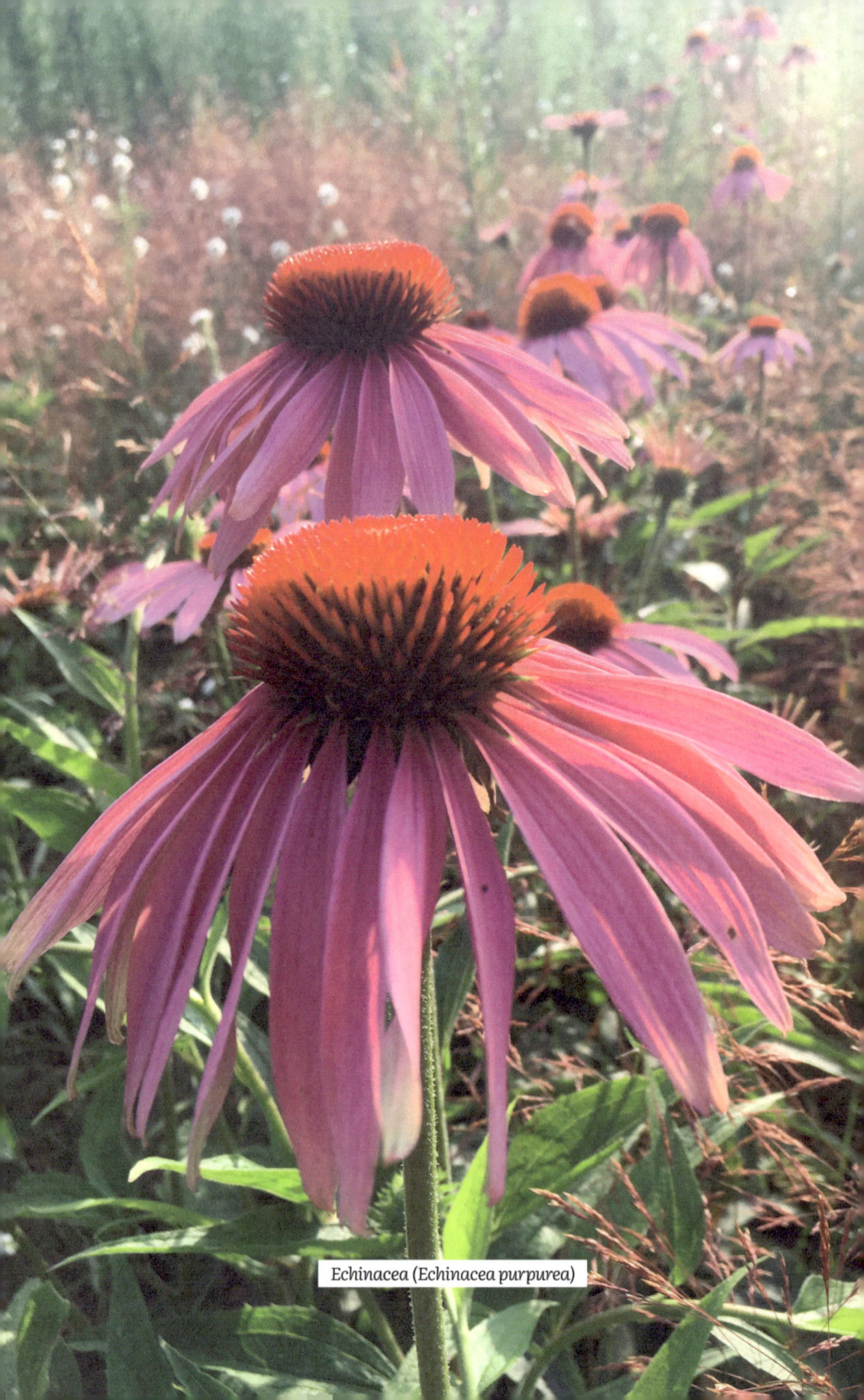
Echinacea (Echinacea purpurea)

CHAPTER 4.
ANTIVIRAL HERBS
(ANTIMICROBIAL)

Antiviral herbs work in a few diverse ways. They can have direct antiviral activity, meaning they inhibit the replication of viruses by interfering with their ability to enter cells, replicate, or assemble new viruses. Included among these are echinacea, garlic, and St. John's wort.

Antiviral herbs can also boost the body's natural immune response, helping it to recognize and eliminate viruses more efficiently. These herbs are known as immunomodulators and include astragalus and ginseng.

Finally, some antiviral herbs have broad-spectrum antimicrobial activity, such as oregano and thyme. With these properties, antiviral herbs can kill a wide variety of microorganisms, including viruses, bacteria, and fungi.

A) Echinacea (Echinacea purpurea)
B) Garlic (Allium sativum)
C) Oregano (Origanum vulgare)
D) Licorice (Glycyrrhiza glabra)
E) Elderflower (Sambucus nigra)
F) Elderberry (Sambucus nigra)
G) St. John's wort (Hypericum perforatum)
H) Astragalus (Astragalus membranaceus)
I) Ginseng (Panax quinquefolius)
J) Thyme (Thyme vulgaris)

Preparation & Dosage

Echinacea (Echinacea purpurea)

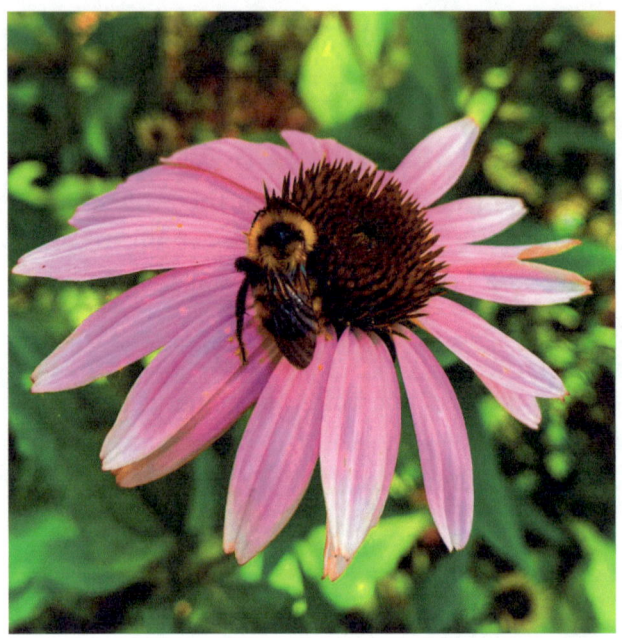

Echinacea is considered an effective antiviral due to its compounds that activate the immune system and enhance the body's natural defenses against viruses. It contains compounds such as polysaccharides, flavonoids, and aklomides that have been shown to have immune-boosting and antiviral properties. The aklomides are also believed to stimulate immune cells such as natural killer cells, while the polysaccharides are thought to activate T cells and B cells that are important in fighting infections. Echinacea is commonly used as an immune-stimulating herb to help support the body's defenses during respiratory viral infections.

Echinacea (Purporea)[1]

Results from clinical studies confirm the antiviral activity found for Echinacea in vitro, embracing enveloped respiratory pathogens and therefore coronaviruses as well. Substantiating results from a new, completed study seem to extrapolate these effects to the prevention of SARS-CoV-2 infections. As hypothesized, the established broad antiviral activity of Echinacea extract appears to be inclusive for SARS-CoV-2.

In 2020, Signer et al. published in vitro data revealing a broad virucidal activity for Echinacea purpurea (hydroethanolic extract (65% v/v) of freshly harvested Echinacea purpurea (L.) Moench (95% aerial parts and 5% root) in pharmaceutical quality according to good manufacturing practices (GMP)) against a broad number of coronaviruses ranging from the typical common cold CoV-229E to highly pathogenic SARS-CoV-2 viruses.

Echinacea Infusion Recipe:

- Add 1 tablespoon of fresh echinacea root OR 2 teaspoons of dried echinacea root to a pot with 2 cups of water.
- Bring to a boil, then turn down the heat to a simmer.
- Simmer for 10 minutes.
- Turn off the heat and steep for 10 minutes.
- Strain and drink up to three times a day.

Echinacea Flower Infusion Recipe:

- Bring 2 cups of water to a boil.
- Add a handful of echinacea flowers and leaves.

---

1 Nicolussi S, Ardjomand-Woelkart K, Stange R, Gancitano G, Klein P, Ogal M. Echinacea as a Potential Force against Coronavirus Infections? A Mini-Review of Randomized Controlled Trials in Adults and Children. *Microorganisms*. 2022; 10(2):211. https://doi.org/10.3390/microorganisms10020211

- Bring the heat down to a simmer and let the herbs simmer for a couple of minutes.
- Turn off heat and steep for 15 minutes.
- Add honey or maple syrup and other aromatic herbs for flavor if desired.
- For a stronger tea, you can use more echinacea flowers.
- Drink a mug of echinacea tea up to three times a day as needed.

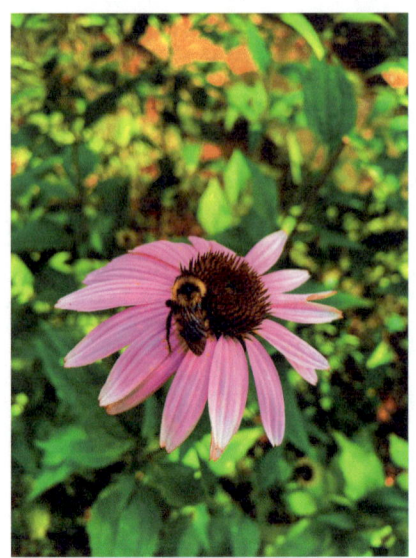

Echinacea Tincture Recipe:

- Chop fresh echinacea root into pieces and place in a jar.
- Pour in enough alcohol to cover, leaving space at the top.*
- Tightly seal the jar, label, date, and shake well.
- Let it steep for 2–3 months. Shake the jar weekly.
- Strain the tincture and store it in a glass bottle.
- Take 10–15 drops diluted in a little bit of water or echinacea tea up to three times a day as needed.
- For children, the proper amount will vary depending on their age and weight. Use 5–7 drops diluted in a small amount of juice or water up to three times a day as needed.

For antiviral purposes, echinacea should be taken at the onset of illness or infection and consistently for up to two weeks afterward.

Note: Echinacea may cause allergic reactions in some people, especially those who have allergies to plants in the Asteraceae family. Echinacea may be contraindicated with certain medications and should not be used by individuals with autoimmune disorders. As with any herbal remedy, it is best to slowly increase the amount used over time and monitor your body's response. Always consult with a clinical herbalist or health care professional before taking herbal remedies, particularly if you have a health-related condition or are taking medication.

Garlic (Allium sativum)

Garlic is considered a strong antiviral due to its high content of sulfur compounds, particularly allicin. Allicin has been shown to have strong antimicrobial and antiviral properties and can help slow down the replication of viruses in the body. Garlic may also help to boost the immune system, strengthening the body's ability to fight off viral infections.

Research has shown that garlic may be effective against a range of viruses, including those that cause the common cold and flu. It can be consumed in a variety of forms to obtain its antiviral benefits, such as raw garlic, cooked garlic, garlic supplements, and garlic extracts.

- Raw Garlic: Eating raw garlic is one of the most effective ways to enjoy its antiviral actions. Simply chop or crush a clove and mix it into a small amount of food.
- Garlic Capsules: Garlic capsules can also be taken as a supplement available at health food stores. Follow the instructions on the package.

Garlic Infusion Recipe:

- Crush 1–2 cloves of garlic.
- Steep in simmering water or chicken bone broth for 5 minutes.
- Strain out the garlic and drink it while it is still warm.

Note: Garlic can be contraindicated with certain medications, including blood thinners and high blood pressure medication. Garlic may also cause gastrointestinal side effects in some individuals, such as heartburn, bloating, and diarrhea. As with any herbal remedy, it is best to slowly increase the amount used over time and monitor your body's response. Always consult with a clinical herbalist or health care professional before taking herbal remedies, particularly if you have a health-related condition or are taking medication.

Oregano (Origanum vulgare)

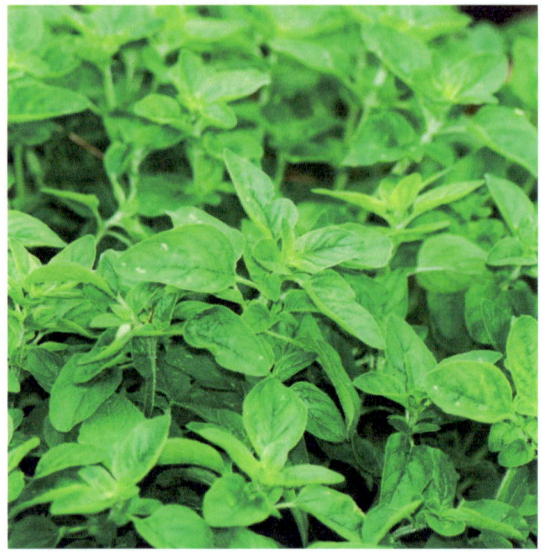

Oregano contains several active compounds, including carvacrol and thymol, that give it its antiviral properties. These compounds have been found to be effective against a wide range of viruses as well as norovirus.

Oregano's antiviral properties are thought to work by disrupting the viral envelope, a protective outer layer that surrounds the virus. By breaking down the viral envelope, oregano prevents the virus from infecting healthy cells and spreading further throughout the body.

It also has immune-boosting properties that can help support the body's defense system against viral infections. Oregano may increase production of white blood cells that fight off infections as well as enhance the activity of natural killer cells and other immune cells.

Overall, the antiviral and immune-boosting properties of oregano make it an effective herb for preventing and treating viral infections. It can be used as an essential oil for topical use or taken as a tea or tincture.

Oregano Infusion Recipe:

- Add 4 teaspoons of fresh oregano leaves OR 2 teaspoons of dried oregano to a cup of hot water.
- Steep for 5 minutes, then strain and drink.
- Add honey or maple syrup and other herbs for flavor if desired.
- Enjoy up to three times a day. For a stronger tea, you can use more oregano leaves.

Oregano Tincture Recipe:

- Fill a jar with dried oregano leaves, leaving some space at the top.
- Pour in enough alcohol to cover, leaving space at the top.*
- Tightly seal the jar, label, date, and shake well.
- Let it steep for 2–3 months. Shake the jar weekly.
- Strain the mixture.
- Store the tincture in a glass jar and label it.
- Take 15 drops diluted in a small amount of water or juice up to three times a day as needed.
- For children, the proper amount will vary depending on their age and weight. Use 5–7 drops diluted in a small amount of juice or water up to three times a day as needed.

Oregano Essential Oil:

Oregano essential oil can be used topically or aromatically to support immune function during viral infections. However, it should be diluted with a carrier oil (10 drops of oregano per ounce of carrier oil) before use, as it can be irritating to the skin.

Note: Oregano can cause gastrointestinal side effects in some individuals such as nausea, vomiting, and diarrhea. Oregano should not be taken in large quantities or for extended periods of time. As with any herbal remedy, it is best to slowly increase the amount used over time and monitor your body's response. Always consult with a clinical herbalist or health care professional before taking herbal remedies, particularly if you have a health-related condition or are taking medication.

Licorice (Glycyrrhiza glabra)

Licorice has been used in TCM for centuries as an antiviral. It contains several compounds, including glycyrrhizin and flavonoids, that give it its antiviral properties. Glycyrrhizin has been found to inhibit the replication of several viruses, including influenza and herpes simplex.

Licorice also has immune-boosting properties that can help to support the body's defense system against viruses. It can also stimulate the production of interferon, a protein that helps to prevent viruses from replicating, as well as enhance the activity of natural killer cells.

Licorice Infusion Recipe:

- Add 4 teaspoons of fresh licorice root OR 2 teaspoons of dried licorice to 2 cups of water.
- Bring to a boil, then turn down to a simmer.
- Simmer for 5–10 minutes, then strain.
- Add lemon and other aromatic herbs for flavor if desired.
- Enjoy up to two times a day. For a stronger tea, use more licorice root.

Licorice Tincture Recipe:

- Chop fresh licorice root into pieces and place in a jar.
- Pour in enough alcohol to cover, leaving space at the top.*
- Tightly seal the jar, label, date, and shake well.
- Let it steep for 2–3 months. Shake the jar weekly.
- Strain the tincture and store it in a glass jar.
- Take 10–15 drops diluted in a little bit of water up to three times a day as needed.
- For children, the proper amount will vary depending on their age and weight. Use 3–5 drops diluted in a small amount of juice or water up to two times a day as needed.

Note: Licorice may have contraindications with certain medications, including blood thinners, blood pressure medications, and some steroids. Licorice may also cause side effects such as hypertension, electrolyte imbalances, and hormonal changes. Licorice should not be taken in copious amounts or for extended periods of time, as it can lead to adverse effects. As with any herbal remedy, it is best to slowly increase the amount used over time and monitor your body's response. Always consult with a clinical herbalist or health care professional before taking herbal remedies, particularly if you have a health-related condition or are taking medication.

Elder Flower (Sambucus nigra)

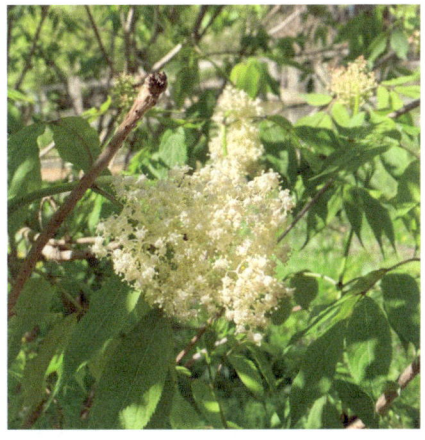

The elderflower has been traditionally used for its immune-boosting properties, particularly for fighting respiratory infections such as colds, flu, and other viruses. The specific mechanisms through which elderflower works to combat these viral infections are still being studied, but there are several potential factors that may contribute to its effectiveness.

- Elderflower compounds have been shown to have antiviral effects against influenza and a range of viruses. They may help to inhibit viral replication and reduce the severity of symptoms.
- These compounds may also reduce inflammation in the respiratory tract and improve breathing. This can be particularly beneficial for individuals with respiratory infections who may experience inflammation in the lungs.
- Elderflowers are believed to have immunostimulant properties, meaning that they enhance the immune system's abilities to fight infections. This can be especially important for those with weakened immune systems who may be more susceptible to viral infections.

Elderflowers have been shown to have mucolytic effects that may help to break down mucus and phlegm in the respiratory tract. This can help alleviate congestion and improve breathing, which can be beneficial for individuals with respiratory infections.

Elderflower Syrup Recipe:

Ingredients:

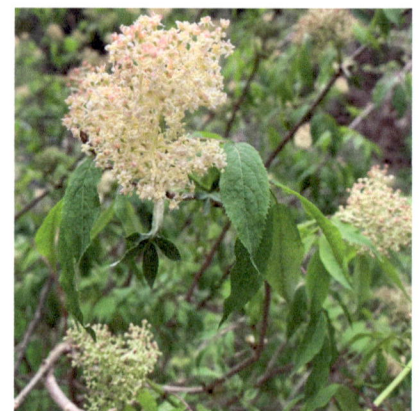

- 2 cups of fresh elderflowers OR 1 cup of dried elderflower
- 4 cups of water
- 2 cups of sugar, maple syrup, or coconut sugar
- Juice of 1 lemon (optional)

Instructions:

- Rinse the elderflowers and remove the thick stems.
- In a pot, bring the water to a boil.

- Add the elderflowers and steep for 30 minutes.
- Strain the flowers through cheesecloth.
- Add the honey or sugar to the liquid and bring to a simmer, stirring until the sweetener is completely dissolved.
- Continue to simmer until about half of the water evaporates.
- Add lemon juice if desired.
- Remove from heat and let cool.
- Pour the syrup into a clean glass jar or bottle and store in the refrigerator.

Dosage:

- Have 1–2 tablespoons of elderflower syrup up to four times a day at first signs of a cold or flu.
- For children over the age of one, give 1–2 teaspoons of elderflower syrup up to four times a day at first signs of a cold or flu.

Note: Elderflower syrup should not be given to children under one year old. Consult with a clinical herbalist or a qualified health care professional before using elderflower syrup if you have health conditions or are taking medications.

Elderflower Infusion Recipe:

- Place 1 tablespoon of fresh elderflowers OR 2 teaspoons of dried elderflowers into a tea ball.
- Place in a mug and pour simmering water over the herbs.
- Steep for 5–10 minutes.
- Add honey and lemon if desired.
- Drink 1–2 cups per day as needed.

Elderflower Tincture Recipe:

- Chop fresh or dried elderflowers and place in a jar.
- Pour in enough alcohol to cover, leaving space at the top.*
- Tightly seal the jar, label, date, and shake well.

- Let it steep for 2–3 months. Shake the jar weekly.
- Strain the tincture.
- Store in a dark place.
- Use 15–20 drops of elderflower tincture up to four times a day as needed.
- For children, the proper amount will vary depending on their age and weight. Use 5–7 drops diluted in a small amount of juice or water up to four times a day as needed.

Note: Always consult with a clinical herbalist or health care professional before taking herbal remedies, particularly if you have a health-related condition or are taking medication.

Elderberry (Sambucus nigra)

Elderberry contains bioactive compounds including a flavonoid called anthocyanin that interferes with the ability of viruses to enter and replicate within host cells. It is an immune-stimulating herb, elderberry is often used to support the immune system during viral infections such as flus and colds. However, elderberry has been traditionally used in some cultures for its diaphoretic properties.

Elderberry Infusion Recipe:

- Place 2–4 teaspoons of fresh elderberries OR 1–2 teaspoons of dried elderberries to a tea ball or tea bag.
- Place in a mug and pour steeping water over the berries.
- Steep for 10–15 minutes.
- Add honey or maple syrup and lemon if desired.
- For a stronger tea, you can use more elderberries.
- Drink 2–3 cups a day as needed.

Elderberry Tincture Recipe:

- Chop fresh or dried elderberries into small pieces and place in a jar.
- Pour in enough alcohol to cover, leaving space at the top.*
- Tightly seal the jar, label, date, and shake well.
- Let it steep for 2–3 months. Shake the jar weekly.
- Strain the tincture and store it in a glass jar.
- Take 10–20 drops diluted in a small amount of water up to four times a day as needed.

For children, the proper amount will vary depending on their age and weight. Use 5–7 drops diluted in a small amount of juice or water up to three times a day as needed.

Elderberry Gummies:

- Elderberry gummies are a convenient and tasty way to consume elderberries.
- The recommended dosage will vary depending on the product, so always follow the instructions on the label.

Note: As with any herbal remedy, it is best to slowly increase the amount used over time and monitor your body's response. Always consult with a clinical herbalist or health care professional before taking herbal remedies, particularly if you have a health-related condition or are taking medication.

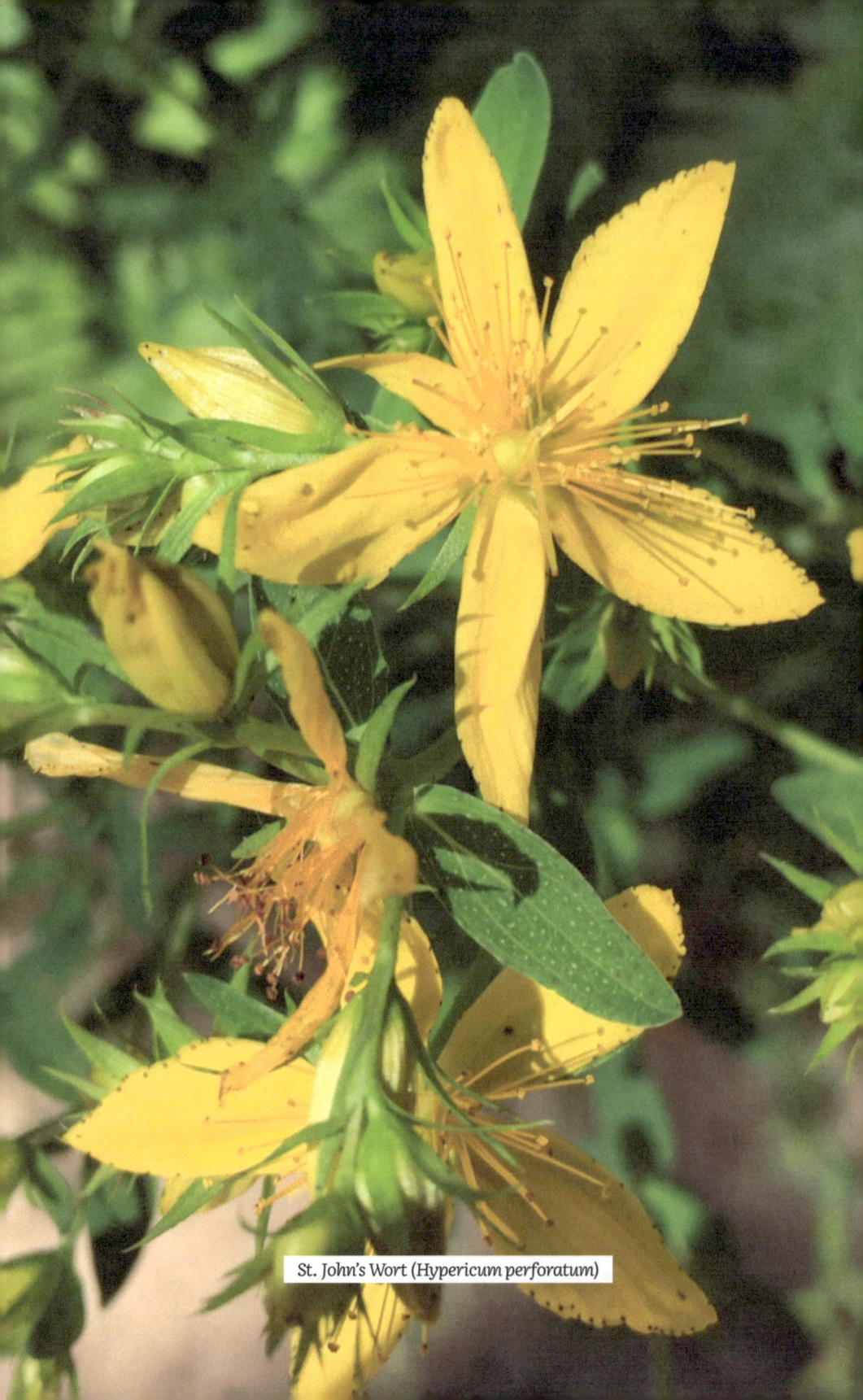

St. John's Wort (*Hypericum perforatum*)

St. John's Wort (Hypericum perforatum)[2]

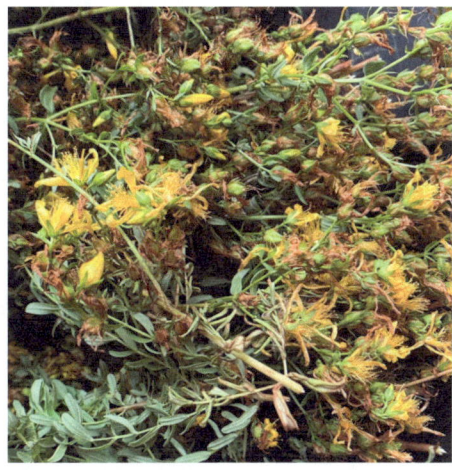

St. John's wort is an herb that supports the respiratory system as an antiviral, expectorant, and anti-inflammatory. Its nervine effects are calming and soothe the discomfort of an illness while fighting the infection (Mcintyre, 1996). When faced with an illness such as the common cold or the flu, add St. John's wort to an herbal blend to strengthen the immune system and protect the respiratory system.

St. John's Wort has been clinically studied for its chemical composition and was proven to be beneficial for its antiviral activities in the infectious bronchitis virus (IBV). The results in the study showed that treatment with H. perforatum significantly reduced the severity of the viral infection. This study confirmed its action and positive results when St. John's wort was extracted in an alcohol tincture.

St. John's Wort Infusion Recipe:

- Place St. John's wort herb in a tea ball or tea bag.
- Place in a mug and pour simmering water over the herbs.
- Steep for 5–10 minutes.
- Add honey or maple syrup and lemon if desired.
- Drink this tea slowly (1 or 2 ounces of tea at a time) and enjoy up to 2 cups per day as needed.

[2] Chen, H., Muhammad, I., Zhang, Y., Ren, Y., Zhang, R., Huang, X., Diao, L., Liu, H., Li, X., Sun, X., Abbas, G., & Li, G. (2019, October 4). *Antiviral Activity Against Infectious Bronchitis Virus and Bioactive Components of Hypericum perforatum L.* Frontiers. https://doi.org/10.3389/fphar.2019.01272

St. John's Wort Tincture Recipe:

- Fill a glass jar about ⅔ full of dried St. John's wort herb.
- Pour in enough alcohol to cover, leaving space at the top.*
- Tightly seal the jar, label, date, and shake well.
- Let it steep for 2–3 months. Shake the jar weekly.
- Strain the tincture into a clean glass jar.
- Take 15 drops diluted in a small amount of water or juice up to three times daily as needed.
- For children, the proper amount will vary depending on their age and weight. Use 5–7 drops diluted in a small amount of juice or water up to three times a day as needed.

Note: St. John's Wort may be contraindicated with certain medications, including antidepressants and birth control pills. Always consult with a clinical herbalist or health care professional before taking herbal remedies, particularly if you have a health-related condition or are taking medication.

Astragalus (Astragalus membranaceus)

Astragalus is an antiviral that supports the immune system in fighting off viral infections. It contains compounds such as polysaccharides, flavonoids, and saponins that have been shown to stimulate the immune system's T cells and natural killer cells. It is thought to activate the production of interferon, a protein that helps prevent viruses from replicating inside cells.

In addition to its antiviral effects, astragalus is also believed to have anti-inflammatory, antioxidant, and cardioprotective effects.

Astragalus Infusion Recipe:

- Bring 2 cups of water to a boil, then lower it to a simmer.
- Add 1–2 teaspoons of dried astragalus root, then cover the pot.
- Simmer for 10 minutes.

- Steep for 5–10 minutes.
- Strain and drink 1–3 cups per day as needed.

Astragalus Tincture Recipe:

- Chop dried astragalus roots into pieces and add to a clean jar.
- Pour in enough alcohol to cover, leaving space at the top.*
- Tightly seal the jar, label, date, and shake well.
- Let it steep for 2–3 months. Shake the jar weekly.
- Strain the mixture, then store it in a glass jar in a dark place.
- Take 15–20 drops of the tincture diluted in water up to three times per day as needed.
- For children, the proper amount will vary depending on their age and weight. Use 5–7 drops diluted in a small amount of juice or water up to three times a day as needed.

Astragalus is considered safe when used appropriately. However, there are some precautions to keep in mind:

- Astragalus may stimulate the immune system, so it should not be used if you have an autoimmune disease or if you are taking immunosuppressant medication.
- Astragalus may be contraindicated with medications that are processed by the liver, so it is best to consult with a clinical herbalist or a qualified health care professional if you are taking any medication that may be affected by liver metabolism.
- Astragalus has the potential to lower blood sugar, so people with diabetes should monitor their blood sugar levels closely and adjust their medication dosage as needed.
- Astragalus may have a diuretic effect, so it is important to stay adequately hydrated when using this herb.

As with any herbal remedy, it is best to slowly increase the amount used over time and monitor your body's response. Always consult with a clinical herbalist or health care professional before taking herbal remedies, particularly if you have a health-related condition or are taking medication.

Ginseng (Panax)

Ginseng contains ginsenosides that are believed to have antiviral properties. These compounds inhibit the ability of viruses to replicate and stimulate the immune system to fight off viral infections. Ginseng has also been found to have anti-inflammatory effects, which may be helpful in reducing the severity of symptoms caused by viral infections.

Ginseng Panax Decoction Recipe:

A decoction is made by boiling the roots of herbs in water for 15 minutes or longer.

- Place 1–2 teaspoons of chopped dried ginseng root in a pot with 2 cups of water.
- Bring the water to a boil.
- Cover the pot.
- Reduce the heat and let it simmer for 20–25 minutes.
- Add natural sweetener or lemon if desired.
- Strain the decoction and drink it warm up to two times a day.

Ginseng Panax Tincture Recipe:

- Chop or grind ¼ to ½ cup of dried ginseng root and put in a jar.
- Pour in enough alcohol to cover, leaving space at the top.*
- Tightly seal the jar, label, date, and shake well.
- Let it steep for 2–3 months. Shake the jar weekly.
- Strain the mixture, then store it in a glass jar in a dark place.
- Take 15–20 drops diluted in water up to three times per day as needed.
- For children, the proper amount will vary depending on their age and weight. Use 5–7 drops diluted in a small amount of juice or water up to three times a day as needed.

Note: Ginseng may be taken for three months at a time. At that point, it is crucial to give yourself a break for a couple of weeks, as prolonged use can lead to side effects. Always consult with a clinical herbalist or health care professional before taking herbal remedies, particularly if you have a health-related condition or are taking medication.

Thyme (Thyme vulgaris)

Thyme contains compounds such as thymol and carvacrol that possess antiviral properties. These compounds can help inhibit the replication of viruses by disrupting their cellular membranes, thus interfering with their ability to enter host cells. Thyme also contains anti-inflammatory and antioxidant flavonoids that support the immune system and reduce inflammation associated with viral infections.

Thyme Infusion Recipe:

- Chop 1 tablespoon of fresh thyme leaves OR 2 teaspoons of dried thyme leaves and stems and place in a tea ball.
- Place in a mug and pour simmering water over the herbs.
- Steep for 10 minutes.
- Add natural sweetener or lemon if desired.
- Drink while warm. Enjoy 2–3 mugs per day as needed.

Thyme Tincture Recipe:

- Rinse 1 cup of fresh thyme leaves OR dried thyme leaves and chop them coarsely.
- Put the thyme leaves in a clean glass jar.
- Pour in enough alcohol to cover, leaving space at the top.*
- Tightly seal the jar, label, date, and shake well.
- Let it steep for 2–3 months. Shake the jar weekly.
- Strain the mixture.
- Squeeze all the liquid out of the tincture using cheesecloth or press it out of the strainer.
- Pour the tincture into glass bottles and store in a dark place.

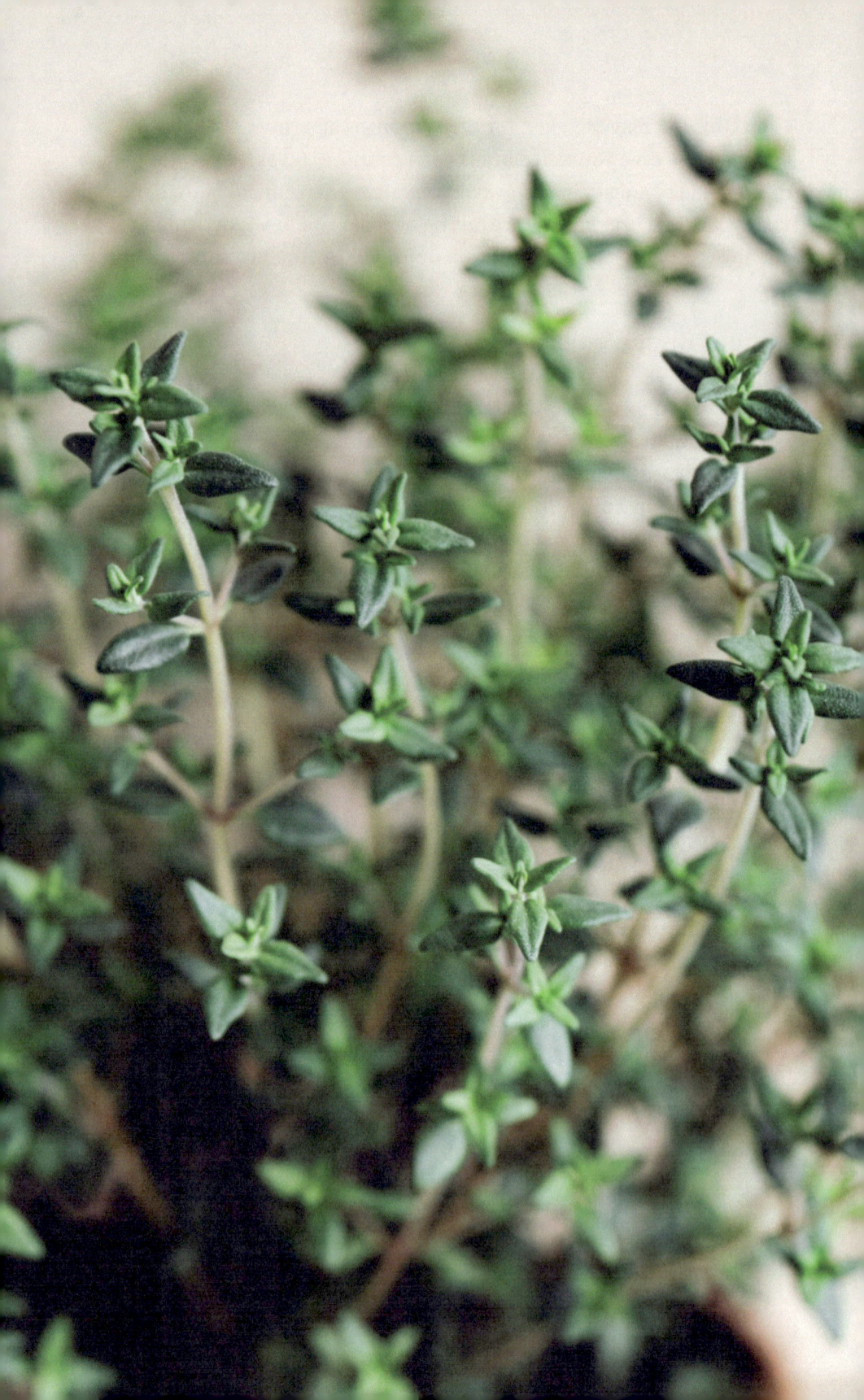

- Take 15 drops diluted in a small amount of water or juice up to three times per day.
- For children, the proper amount will vary depending on their age and weight. Use 5–7 drops diluted in a small amount of juice or water up to three times a day as needed.

Note: It is important to note that thyme tincture should not be used during pregnancy or breastfeeding and may interact with certain medications. Always consult with a clinical herbalist or health care professional before taking herbal remedies, particularly if you have a health-related condition or are taking medication.

Here are some additional ways to enjoy the benefits of thyme:

Topical Thyme Rub:

- Dilute thyme oil with virgin coconut oil or olive oil before applying it to the skin. (Use 10 drops of thyme oil to an ounce of carrier oil.)
- Apply the mixture to the affected area and massage gently.

Thyme Steam Vapor:

- Add a few drops of thyme oil to a bowl of simmering water.
- Cover your head and the bowl with a towel and breathe the steam in deeply.

Aromatherapy:

- Add a few drops of thyme oil to an oil burner or diffuser to release the aroma into the air.
- Close your eyes and take a deep breath of the vapor.
- Continue to diffuse the room you are staying in and breathe in the aroma in the atmosphere.
- Occasionally take a deeper breath of the vapor.

Note: Thyme oil is potent and should always be diluted before use. Additionally, some people may be allergic or sensitive to thyme oil and should avoid using it. If you experience any adverse reactions, it is recommended to consult with a clinical herbalist or a qualified health care professional for any concerns.

Antiviral Food & Recipes

Whole Foods to Eat During a Viral Infection:

There are many whole foods that can help boost the immune system and fight viral infections.

- Citrus fruits are a natural source of vitamin C, which supports the immune system's response to increase the production of white blood cells that fight infections.
- Garlic has antiviral and antibacterial properties.
- Ginger contains gingerol, which has antiviral and antibacterial properties.
- Berries are high in mucilage and vitamin C, supporting a boost in the immune system.
- Leafy greens are high in nutrients including vitamin C and antioxidants that can help fight infections.
- Nuts and seeds are high in vitamin E, an antioxidant that helps boost the immune system.
- Lean proteins such as chicken, turkey, and fish are high in zinc and nutrients that can help fight infections.
- Whole grains are high in vitamins, minerals, and fiber, which support the immune system and overall health.

Consuming a wide variety of foods is necessary to balance your diet and ensure you are getting all the necessary nutrients to best support your immune system.

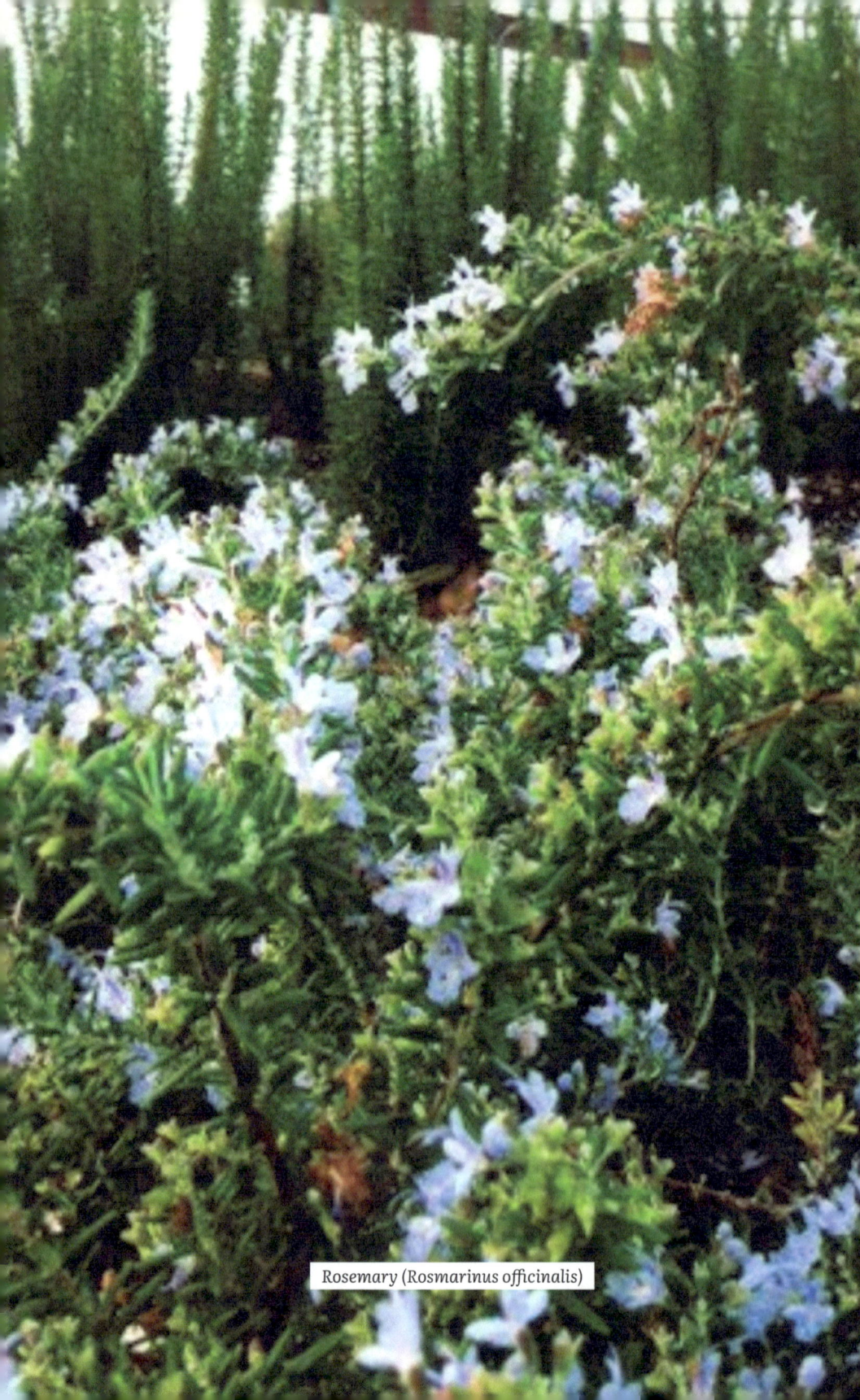

Rosemary (Rosmarinus officinalis)

CHAPTER 5.
ASTRINGENT HERBS

Herbal astringents work by tightening and toning the tissue they come into contact with. They are rich in tannins, naturally occurring polyphenols that can bind with and precipitate proteins. This results in the tissue shrinking or contracting, which can help to reduce inflammation, soothe irritation, and promote healing. This action also reduces swelling in tissue and blood vessels, which can help to reduce bleeding.

Herbal astringents have different actions on the lungs, intestines, swollen glands, and lymph nodes. For the lungs, astringents support the reduction of inflammation and irritation of the respiratory tract, which can improve breathing and alleviate symptoms such as coughing and wheezing.

For the intestines, astringents may help reduce inflammation and irritation in the digestive tract. This helps to improve digestion and alleviates symptoms such as cramping and diarrhea.

For swollen glands and lymph nodes, by helping to tighten and tone the tissues in the affected area, astringents reduce inflammation and support the natural healing processes.

Additionally, some astringent herbs have antimicrobial properties that can fight off infections that may be causing the swelling in the first place. Overall, the actions of astringent herbs can help to support the lymphatic system that often becomes overwhelmed during periods of infection or inflammation, which plays a key role in immune function.

The specific effects of astringent herbs vary depending on the plant and its unique chemical constituents.

Intestinal Astringents:

A) Slippery elm (Ulmus fulva)
B) Marshmallow (Althaea officinalis)
C) Meadowsweet (Filipendula ulmaria)
D) Goldenseal (Hydrastis canadensis)
E) Blackberry (Rubus spp.)
F) Oak bark (Quercus spp.)
G) Plantain (Plantago spp.)

Preparation & Dosage

Slippery Elm (Ulmus fulva)

Slippery elm, an herb used as an astringent to help tighten and soothe the digestive tract, is commonly used for treatment of the intestines. Leaky gut syndrome may occur from a viral infection that enters the circulatory system and causes sepsis, resulting in serious illnesses. Slippery elm is one effective treatment and a potential cure for such conditions.

Slippery Elm Slurry Recipe:

- Add 2 teaspoons of slippery elm powder into a mug.
- Add simmering water and mix.
- Steep for 5–10 minutes.
- Add honey or maple syrup and other herbs for aromatic flavor if desired.
- For a stronger tea, you can use more slippery elm powder.
- Drink a mug up to three times a day between meals as needed.

Slippery elm lozenges can be sucked on to soothe sore throats and coughs.

Note: Drink plenty of water when consuming slippery elm, as it can absorb water and form a gel-like substance in the digestive tract.

Note: Slippery elm may be contraindicated with certain medications including blood thinners and some medications for diabetes and high blood pressure. Slippery elm may also cause nausea, vomiting, and allergic reactions in some individuals. As with any herbal remedy, it is best to slowly increase the amount used over time and monitor your body's response. Always consult with a clinical herbalist or health care professional before taking herbal remedies, particularly if you have a health-related condition or are taking medication.

Marshmallow (Althea officinalis)

Marshmallow is an herb commonly used as a demulcent. However, it can also be blended with astringent herbs to help soothe the intestines.

Marshmallow Infusion Recipe:

- Add 2 teaspoons of dried marshmallow root into a mug.
- Pour simmering water over the herbs.
- Steep for 5–10 minutes, then strain.
- Add honey or maple syrup and lemon (or other herbs for flavor) if desired.
- Enjoy up to four times a day. For a stronger tea, you can use more marshmallow root.

All the mallow species are astringents that will soothe and tighten the intestines. The mucilaginous benefits across the variants are the same.

Marshmallow Capsules:

- Marshmallow capsules are also available at health food stores. Follow the directions for usage on the package.
- Capsules typically contain dried marshmallow root extract and may be standardized to a certain concentration of mucilage.

Note: Marshmallow may be contraindicated with certain medications including blood thinners and some medications for diabetes and high blood pressure. Marshmallows may also cause nausea, vomiting, and allergic reactions in some people. As with any herbal remedy, it is best to slowly increase the amount used over time and monitor your body's response. Always consult with a clinical herbalist or health care professional before taking herbal remedies, particularly if you have a health-related condition or are taking medication.

Meadowsweet (Filipendula ulmaria)

Meadowsweet contains tannins that give it astringent properties when consumed. The tannins bind to proteins in the tissues of the body, causing them to tighten and constrict. This can help to reduce inflammation and irritation as well as reduce excess secretions in the body. Additionally, meadowsweet contains salicylic acid, an anti-inflammatory with pain relieving effects.

Meadowsweet Infusion Recipe:

- Place 1–2 teaspoons of dried meadowsweet flowers and leaves in a tea ball.
- Place in a mug and pour simmering water over the herbs.
- Steep for 5–10 minutes.
- Add honey or other herbs for flavor if desired.
- For a stronger tea, you can use increase the amount of meadowsweet.

- Sip on the tea throughout the day between meals. Drink about an ounce at a time for efficient absorption into the tissue.

Meadowsweet Tincture Recipe:

- Put dried meadowsweet herb in a glass jar.
- Pour in enough alcohol to cover, leaving space at the top.*
- Tightly seal the jar, label, date, and shake well.
- Let it steep for 2–3 months. Shake the jar weekly.
- Strain the liquid through cheesecloth or strainer and transfer the tincture to a clean glass jar.
- Store the tincture in a cool place.
- Take 10–20 drops diluted in a small amount of water or juice up to three times a day as needed.
- For children, the proper amount will vary depending on their age and weight. Use 5–7 drops diluted in a small amount of juice or water up to three times a day as needed.

Note: Meadowsweet may be contraindicated with blood thinners, some diabetic medications, and for people with high blood pressure. Meadowsweet may also cause uncomfortable side effects such as stomachaches and allergic reactions in some individuals. As with any herbal remedy, it is best to slowly increase the amount used over time and monitor your body's response. Always consult with a clinical herbalist or health care professional before taking herbal remedies, particularly if you have a health-related condition or are taking medication.

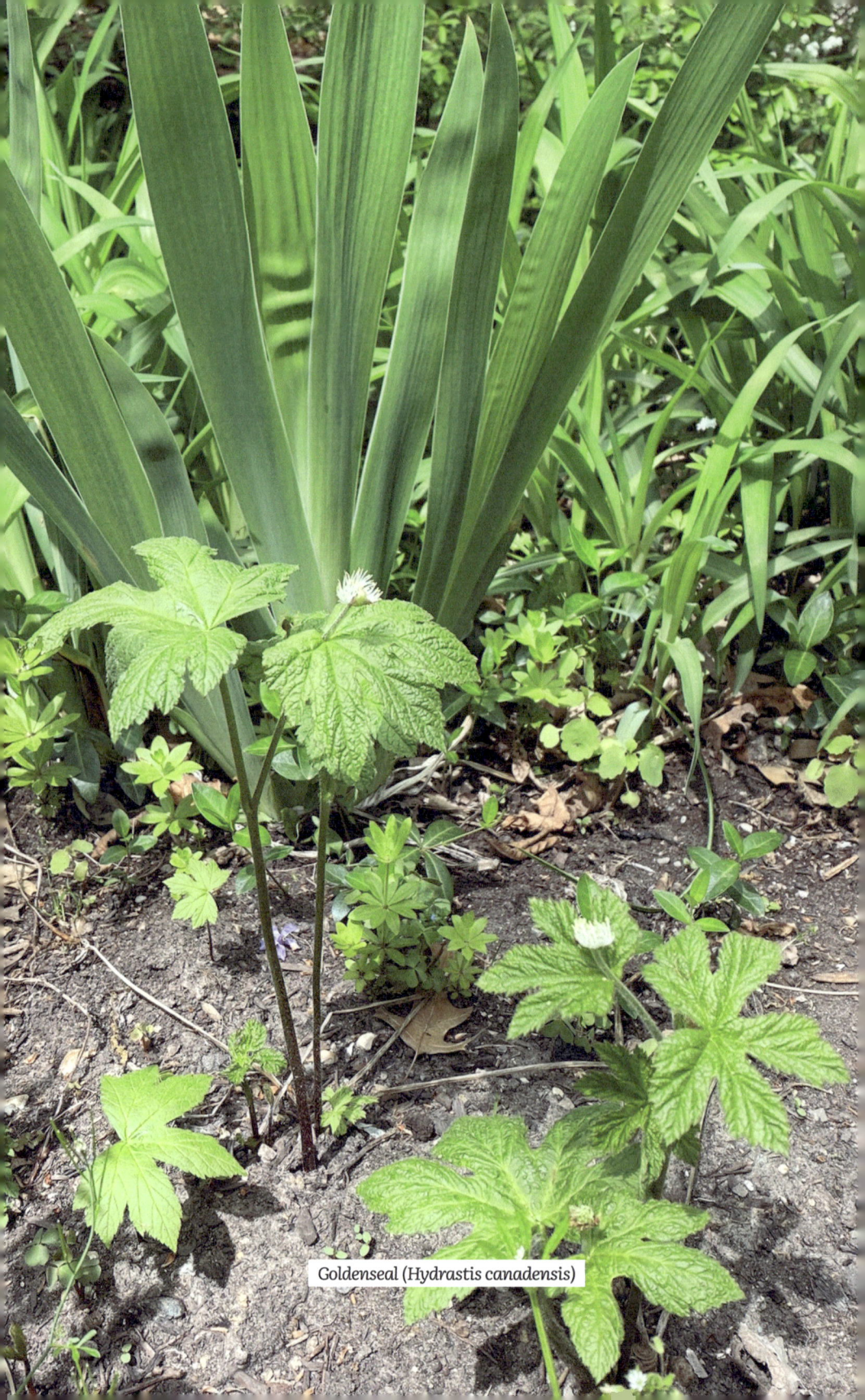
Goldenseal (Hydrastis canadensis)

Goldenseal (Hydrastis canadensis)

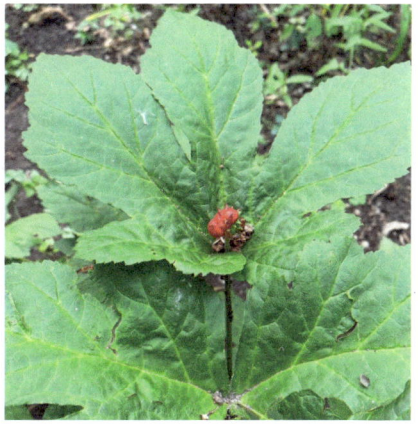

Goldenseal contains berberine, an astringent compound that has positive effects on the digestive system. When ingested, berberine can help to tighten and tone the mucous membranes in the digestive tract, reduce inflammation, and mend raw tissues. This can be helpful in treating conditions such as gastritis, diarrhea, and ulcerative colitis where there is inflammation and irritation in the digestive tract. Additionally, goldenseal has antimicrobial properties that may help to prevent and strengthen the immune system to fight infections in the digestive tract.

Goldenseal Decoction Recipe:

- Add 2 teaspoons of dried goldenseal root to a pot with 2 cups of water.
- Bring to a boil, then cover the pot.
- Simmer for 15–20 minutes.
- Strain the mixture.
- Add a natural sweetener and other aromatic herbs for flavor if desired.
- Drink up to three mugs of tea a day as needed between meals.

Goldenseal Capsules:

- This herb is also available in capsule form in health food stores. Follow directions for use on the package.
- Capsules typically contain dried goldenseal root extract and may be standardized to a certain concentration of berberine.

Note: Goldenseal may be contraindicated for certain medications such as blood thinners, antibiotics, and some of the medications for heart disease and high blood pressure. Goldenseal may also cause side effects in some people such as stomachaches and allergic reactions. As with any herbal remedy, it is best to slowly increase the amount used over time and monitor your body's response. Always consult with a clinical herbalist or health care professional before taking herbal remedies, particularly if you have a health-related condition or are taking medication.

Blackberry (Rubus spp.)

Blackberry leaves and berries are astringent due to their high tannin content. Tannins are naturally occurring plant compounds that have a drying and tightening effect on tissues, making them useful for reducing inflammation, soothing irritation, and improving wound healing. As a result, blackberry leaves and fruit help slow down the flow of diarrhea.

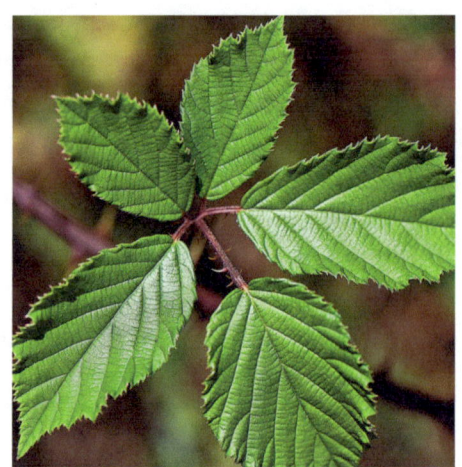

Blackberry Infusion Recipe:

- Put 1–2 teaspoons of dried blackberry leaves into a tea ball.
- Place in a mug and pour simmering water over the herbs.
- Steep for 5–10 minutes.
- You can also use the berries either fresh or dried. If using blackberries instead of leaves, steep 1–2 tablespoons of the fruit in hot water for 10–15 minutes.
- Drink an ounce at a time between meals. Enjoy up to three cups a day as needed.

Blackberry Syrup Recipe:

Ingredients:

- 2 cups fresh or frozen blackberries
- 1 cup water
- 1 cup honey
- 1 tablespoon lemon juice
- 1 teaspoon grated ginger (optional)

Instructions:

- In a saucepan, combine the blackberries and water. Bring to a boil and then reduce heat to a simmer.
- Let simmer for 10–15 minutes, stirring occasionally. Let the blackberries cook down and reduce the liquid.
- Remove from heat and let cool.
- Strain the mixture through cheesecloth, pressing the blackberries to extract as much liquid as possible. Discard the seeds.
- Return the liquid to the saucepan and add honey, lemon juice, and grated ginger (optional). Stir well to combine.
- Bring the mixture back to a simmer, then cook for 10–15 minutes, stirring occasionally, until the syrup has thickened slightly.
- Remove from heat and let cool.
- Pour into a glass jar with a tight-fitting lid.
- Refrigerate for up to three months.
- Take 1–2 tablespoons up to three times a day as needed.
- For children, the proper amount will vary depending on their age and weight. Use 1–2 teaspoons up to three times a day as needed.

Blackberry syrup is also available commercially.

Note: Blackberries may be contraindicated with certain medications such as blood thinners and may cause stomachaches and allergic reactions in some individuals. As with any herbal remedy, it is best to slowly increase the amount used over time and monitor your body's response. Always consult with a clinical herbalist or health care professional before taking herbal remedies, particularly if you have a health-related condition or are taking medication.

Oak Bark (Quercus spp.)

Oak bark contains astringent compounds such as tannins and catechins that can tighten and tone tissues. When used topically, oak bark can help to constrict blood vessels and reduce inflammation. It produces a similar effect on the digestive system when taken internally, helping to reduce inflammation and diarrhea. Overall, oak bark is a powerful astringent that supports a healthy digestive system.

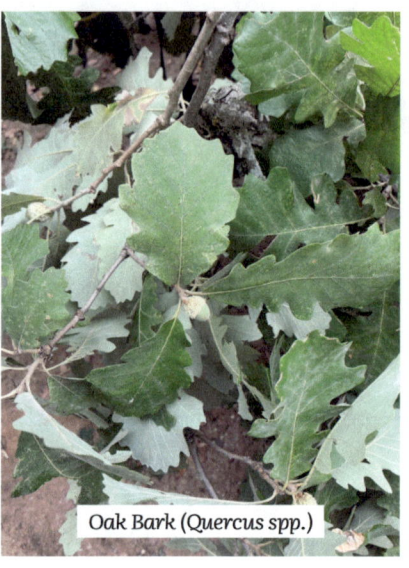

Oak Bark (Quercus spp.)

Oak Bark Decoction Recipe:

- Add 2 tablespoons of dried oak bark to a pot with 2 cups of water.
- Bring to a boil, then lower the heat and simmer for 10–20 minutes.
- Remove from the heat.
- Strain the mixture.
- Add natural sweetener and lemon (or other herbs for flavor) if desired.
- Enjoy up to two times per day (or once for children). For a stronger tea, use more oak bark.

Oak Bark Tincture Recipe:

- Place dried oak bark in a clean glass jar.
- Pour in enough alcohol to cover, leaving space at the top.*
- Tightly seal the jar, label, date, and shake well.

- Let it steep for 2–3 months. Shake the jar weekly.
- Strain the mixture through cheesecloth.
- Store the tincture in a glass jar, in a cool place.
- Take 10–20 drops diluted with a little bit of water up to three times a day as needed.
- For children, the proper amount will vary depending on their age and weight. Use 5–7 drops diluted in a small amount of juice or water up to three times a day as needed.

Note: Oak bark may be contraindicated for certain medications, including blood thinners and some medications for high blood pressure. Oak bark may also cause stomachaches and allergic reactions in some individuals. As with any herbal remedy, it is best to slowly increase the amount used over time and monitor your body's response. Always consult with a clinical herbalist or health care professional before taking herbal remedies, particularly if you have a health-related condition or are taking medication.

Plantain (Plantago spp.)

Plantains have a high mucilage content, making them soothing and healing to irritated mucous membranes. The tannins found in plantains give them astringent properties that help to tighten and tone tissues. Plantain makes an excellent treatment for diarrhea and hemorrhoids due to its strong astringent and anti-inflammatory properties.

Plantain Infusion Recipe:

- Place a handful of fresh plantain leaves OR 2 tablespoons of dried plantain leaves to a mug.
- Pour simmering water over the herbs.
- Steep for 5–10 minutes, then strain.
- Add honey or maple syrup and lemon (or other herbs for flavor) if desired.
- For a stronger tea, you can use more plantain.
- Drink 2–3 mugs a day, sipping an ounce at a time, as needed.

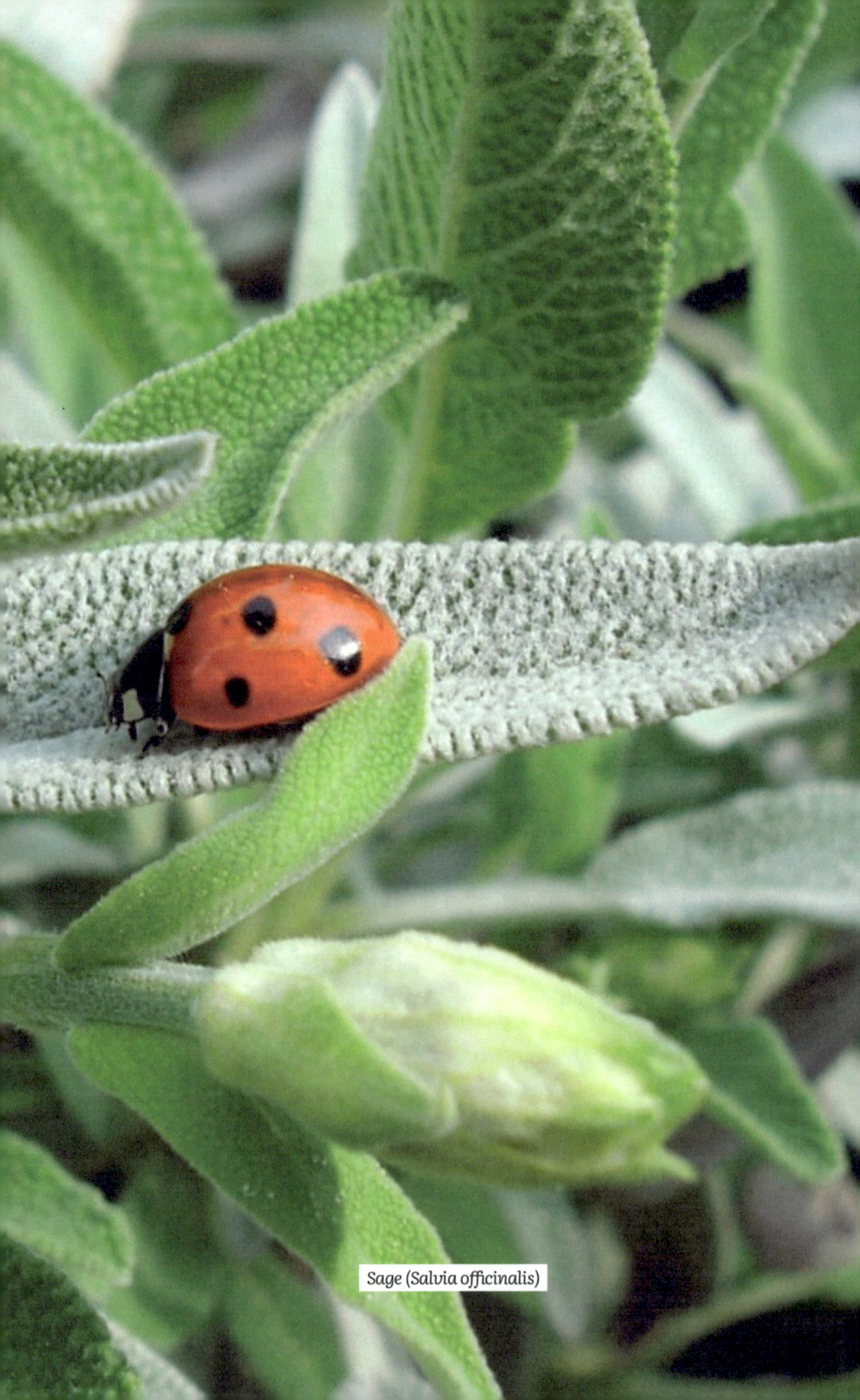
Sage (Salvia officinalis)

Plantain Tincture Recipe:

- Chop or grind dried plantain leaves and place them in a jar.
- Pour in enough alcohol to cover, leaving space at the top.*
- Tightly seal the jar, label, date, and shake well.
- Let it steep for 2–3 months. Shake the jar weekly.
- Strain the mixture, then store it in a glass jar in a dark place.
- Take 10–20 drops diluted in a little bit of water up to three times a day.
- For children, the proper amount will vary depending on their age and weight. Use 5–7 drops diluted in a small amount of juice or water up to three times a day as needed.

Note: As with any herbal remedy, it is best to slowly increase the amount used over time and monitor your body's response. Always consult with a clinical herbalist or health care professional before taking herbal remedies, particularly if you have a health-related condition or are taking medication.

Lung Astringents:

In the lungs, astringents can help reduce inflammation and irritation of the respiratory tract, which can improve breathing as well as alleviate symptoms such as coughing, wheezing, and congestion from colds, flu, and viruses.

A) Sage (Salvia officinalis)
B) Rosemary (Rosmarinus officinalis)
C) Oregano (Origanum vulgare)
D) Thyme (Thymus vulgaris)
E) Elecampane (Inula Helenium)
F) Plantain (Plantago spp.)

Sage (Salvia officinalis)

Sage is an astringent herb for various respiratory conditions, including coughs, bronchitis, and sore throats. It contains essential oils, flavonoids, and tannins that give it its astringent properties.

Sage works as an astringent for the lungs by toning and strengthening the tissues of the respiratory tract. The tannins in sage help to tighten and constrict the tissues, thus reducing inflammation and preventing excessive mucus production. Its essential oils also have antiseptic and antibacterial compounds that can help to clear infections and promote healing in the respiratory tract.

This combination of properties makes sage a useful herb for promoting respiratory health and providing relief from respiratory symptoms.

Sage Infusion Recipe:

- Put 1–2 teaspoons of dried sage leaves into a tea ball or tea bag.
- Place in a mug and pour simmering water over the herbs.
- Steep for 5–10 minutes.
- Add honey or maple syrup and lemon (other aromatic herbs for flavor) if desired.
- Enjoy up to three times a day (or two for children). For a stronger tea, you can use more sage.

Sage Tincture Recipe:

- Put fresh sage leaves or dried sage leaves in a glass jar.
- Pour in enough alcohol to cover, leaving space at the top.*
- Tightly seal the jar, label, date, and shake well.
- Let it steep for 2–3 months. Shake the jar weekly.
- Strain the tincture through cheesecloth, pressing the leaves to extract all the liquid.
- Transfer the tincture to a glass jar and store in a dark place.

- Take 7–10 drops diluted in a small amount of water or juice up to three times a day as needed.
- For children, the proper amount will vary depending on their age and weight. Use 3–5 drops diluted in a small amount of juice or water up to three times a day as needed.

Note: As with any herbal remedy, it is best to slowly increase the amount used over time and monitor your body's response. Always consult with a clinical herbalist or health care professional before taking herbal remedies, particularly if you have a health-related condition or are taking medication.

Sage Steam Vapor:

- Boil a pot of water, remove from heat, and add a cup of fresh or dried sage leaves.
- Drape a towel over the bowl and your head, taking deep breaths of the steam for 5–10 minutes.
- Do this as often as needed until you feel some relief, about three times a day.

Aromatherapy Diffuser:

- Add sage essential oil to a diffuser and breathe in the vapors.
- Leave the diffuser running to purify the air and help clear the air passages so you can breathe through your nose.
- Occasionally take a deep breath of the vapors.
- Adjust how often you deep breathe in the vapors based on how you feel.

Note: Sage may be contraindicated with certain medications, including blood thinners and medications for diabetes and high blood pressure. Sage may also cause stomachaches and allergic reactions in some individuals. As with any herbal remedy, it is best to slowly increase the amount used over time and monitor your body's response. Always consult with a clinical herbalist or health care professional before taking herbal remedies, particularly if you have a health-related condition or are taking medication.

Rosemary (Rosmarinus officinalis)

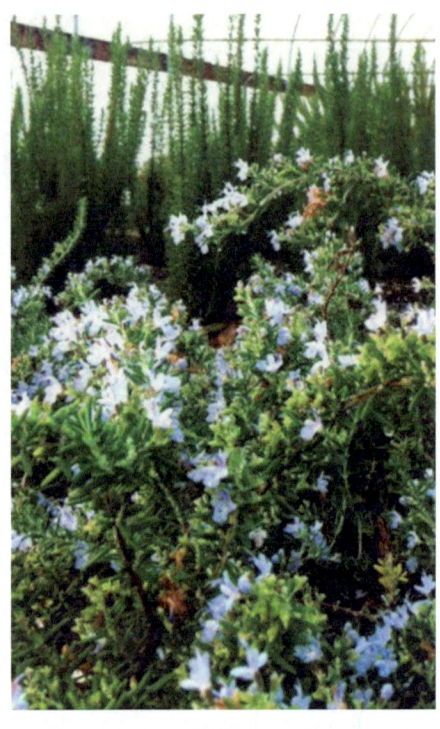

Rosemary's expectorant properties help to loosen and expel mucus from the lungs, making it easier to breathe. Additionally, its anti-inflammatory compounds reduce inflammation in the lungs, airways, and the body in general, while its astringent properties reduce inflammation in the digestive tract. Rosemary's anti-inflammatory actions have even been found to be helpful as an analgesic.

As a carminative, rosemary may help soothe the digestive system and reduce gas and bloating. Its antioxidant compounds, rosmarinic acid and carnosic acid, are antioxidants that may protect the body from free radical damage. Additionally, it contains compounds such as cineole and camphor with antimicrobial properties that may help fight off infections.

Beyond its physical effects, rosemary is known for its calming nervine effect on the nervous system, which may help reduce stress and anxiety. Rosemary can also help improve blood flow and circulation in the body.

Overall, rosemary is a versatile herb that can be used as an herbal remedy for a wide range of health conditions, including digestive issues, inflammation, infections, and stress.

Rosemary Infusion Recipe:

- Place a generous amount (about a handful) of fresh rosemary sprigs OR 3 tablespoons of dried rosemary in a pot with 2 cups of water.
- Bring to a boil, reduce the heat, and simmer for 2–5 minutes.
- Remove from heat and steep for 5–10 minutes.
- Add natural sweetener and lemon for flavor if desired.
- Slowly sip up to three cups a day as needed.
- For a stronger tea, you can use more rosemary.

Rosemary Tincture Recipe:

- Fill a glass jar about ⅔ full of rosemary leaves.
- Pour in enough alcohol to cover, leaving space at the top.*
- Tightly seal the jar, label, date, and shake well.
- Let it steep for 2–3 months. Shake the jar weekly.
- Strain the liquid through cheesecloth or a fine-mesh strainer. Squeeze the rosemary in the cheesecloth to extract as much liquid as possible, then discard the plant material.
- Store in a glass jar in a dark place.
- Take 5–7 drops diluted with a little bit of water or juice up to three times per day as needed.
- For children, the proper amount will vary depending on their age and weight. Use 3–5 drops diluted in a small amount of juice or water up to two times a day as needed.

Note: Rosemary may be contraindicated with certain medications, including blood thinners. It may also cause stomachaches and allergic reactions in some individuals. As with any herbal remedy, it is best to slowly increase the amount used over time and monitor your body's response. Always consult with a clinical herbalist or health care professional before taking herbal remedies, particularly if you have a health-related condition or are taking medication.

Oregano (Origanum vulgare)

Oregano is a powerful astringent and anti-inflammatory often used for treating the lungs. It contains carvacrol and terpenes that help the lungs by reducing congestion, improving airflow, wiping out viruses, cleansing the lungs.

Oregano is a versatile herb with many herbal actions. It supports respiratory health by acting as an expectorant, helping to loosen and expel mucus from the lungs. With its potent antimicrobial properties, oregano can help fight off harmful bacteria, viruses, and fungi in the body, and it also contains antioxidants that help protect the body, relieve inflammation, and oxidative stress. Lastly, oregano contains compounds that may help reduce inflammation, helping to relieve conditions such as inflammatory disorders.

Oregano Infusion Recipe:

- Put 1–2 teaspoons of dried oregano leaves in a tea ball or tea bag.
- Place in a mug and pour simmering water over the herbs.
- Steep for 5–10 minutes.
- Add honey or other herbs for flavor if desired.
- For a stronger tea, you can use more oregano.
- Drink 2–3 cups a day as needed.

Oregano Tincture Recipe:

- Clean and chop either fresh or dried oregano leaves into small pieces and place in a jar.
- Fill the glass jar with the chopped oregano, leaving about ⅓ of the jar empty.
- Pour in enough alcohol to cover, leaving space at the top.*
- Tightly seal the jar, label, date, and shake well.
- Let it steep for 2–3 months. Shake the jar weekly.
- Strain the extract through cheesecloth.
- Store in a clean glass jar in a dark place.

- Take 7–10 drops diluted with a little water up to three times a day as needed.
- For children, the proper amount will vary depending on their age and weight. Use 3–5 drops diluted in a small amount of juice or water up to three times a day as needed.

Oregano Steam Vapor:

- Boil a pot of water, remove from heat, and add a couple of handfuls of fresh or dried oregano leaves.
- Drape a towel over your head and lean over the pot, taking deep breaths of steam for 5–10 minutes up to 3 times a day.

Note: As with any herbal remedy, it is best to slowly increase the amount used over time and monitor your body's response. Always consult with a clinical herbalist or health care professional before taking herbal remedies, particularly if you have a health-related condition or are taking medication.

Thyme (Thymus vulgaris)

As an astringent, thyme helps to tighten and tone tissues, reducing inflammation and promoting healing. This makes thyme a helpful remedy for sore throats, inflamed gums, swollen glands, lymph nodes, irritated lungs, and other conditions affecting the mucous membranes.

As an antiseptic, thyme contains compounds such as thymol and carvacrol that have antibacterial, anti-microbial, and antifungal properties. These properties can be useful for treating respiratory infections as well as bacterial skin infections or fungal infections.

As an antiviral, thyme has been found to be effective against several viruses, including colds, influenza, and herpes simplex virus, as it supports the immune system during viral infections.

As an expectorant, thyme helps to loosen and expel mucus from the respiratory tract. This action may be helpful for coughs, bronchitis, and pneumonia.

Thyme Infusion Recipe:

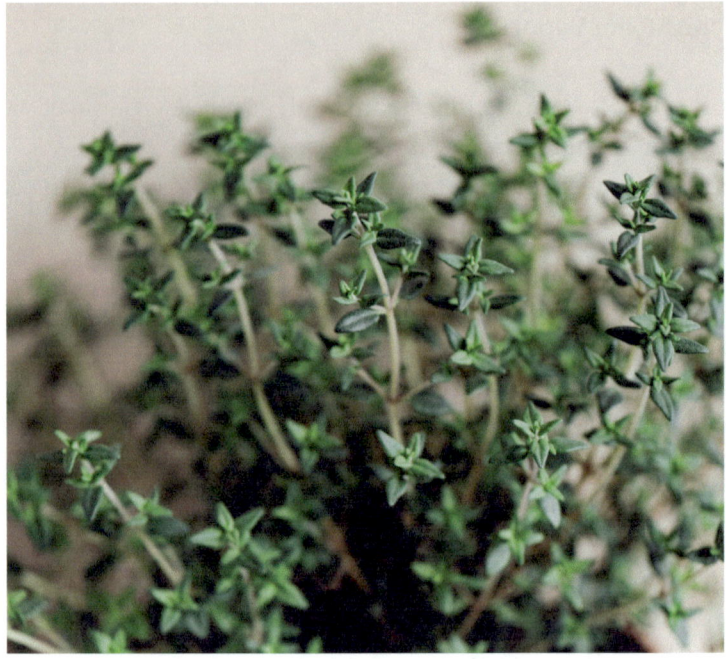

- Cut a handful of fresh thyme OR 2-3 tablespoons of dried thyme and place in a tea ball.
- Place in a mug and pour simmering water over the herbs.
- Steep for 5 minutes if using fresh thyme; steep for 5-10 minutes for dried thyme.
- Add honey or other herbs for flavor if desired.
- For a stronger tea, you can use more thyme.
- Drink 1-2 cups per day as needed.

Thyme Tincture Recipe:

- Fill a clean glass jar with dried thyme leaves.
- Pour in enough alcohol to cover, leaving space at the top.*

- Tightly seal the jar, label, date, and shake well.
- Let it steep for 2–3 months. Shake the jar weekly.
- Strain the tincture through cheesecloth.
- Store in a clean jar in a dark place.
- Take 3–5 drops diluted in a small amount of water or juice up to three times a day as needed.
- For children, use 3 drops diluted in a small amount of juice or water up to two times a day as needed.

Note: Thyme tincture may be contraindicated with certain medications and may cause side effects such as stomachaches and allergic reactions in some individuals. As with any herbal remedy, it is best to slowly increase the amount used over time and monitor your body's response. Always consult with a clinical herbalist or health care professional before taking herbal remedies, particularly if you have a health-related condition or are taking medication.

Elecampane (Inula helenium)

Elecampane is an herb with several medicinal properties that is used to treat various health conditions. It has astringent properties that ease diarrhea and other digestive issues by reducing inflammation and promoting healing, but it is also known to have expectorant properties that help clear congestion in the respiratory system. It helps to loosen and expel mucus from the nasal passages, swollen glands, the lungs, and bronchial tubes, making it easier to breathe.

Elecampane has antimicrobial properties that make it effective against various types of bacteria and fungi as well. It has been traditionally used as an herbal remedy for respiratory infections such as bronchitis and pneumonia. Elecampane can also act as a diaphoretic, meaning it can help promote sweating and increase body temperature to fight off infections and promote detoxification. Lastly, elecampane is considered a general tonic herb that may help strengthen the immune system and promote overall health and well-being.

With a wide range of actions, elecampane is a potent herbal remedy that may be used to treat many health conditions, especially those related to the respiratory and digestive systems.

Elecampane Infusion Recipe:

- Put 1–2 teaspoons of elecampane root in a pot with 2 cups of water.
- Bring to a boil, then reduce the heat and let simmer for 5–10 minutes.
- Strain the mixture.
- Add honey or other herbs for flavor if desired.
- Enjoy up to two times a day (or once a day for children). For a stronger tea, you can use more elecampane.

Elecampane Tincture Recipe:

- Chop or grind the elecampane root and put it in a glass jar.
- Pour in enough alcohol to cover, leaving space at the top.*
- Tightly seal the jar, label, date, and shake well.
- Let it steep for 2–3 months. Shake the jar weekly.
- Strain the mixture through cheesecloth.
- Store the tincture in a glass jar in a dark place.
- Take 5–10 drops diluted in a small amount of water up to three times a day.
- For children, the proper amount will vary depending on their age and weight. Use 5–7 drops diluted in a small amount of juice or water up to three times a day as needed.

Note: Elecampane may interact with certain medications and cause stomachaches and allergic reactions in some individuals. As with any herbal remedy, it is best to slowly increase the amount used over time and monitor your body's response. Always consult with a clinical herbalist or health care professional before taking herbal remedies, particularly if you have a health-related condition or are taking medication.

Plantain (Plantago spp.)

Plantains have astringent properties that help dry up excess mucus secretions in the respiratory tract and digestive system. Traditionally, it has been used as an herbal remedy for colds and diarrhea. Plantain has several herbal actions, including astringent, demulcent, anti-inflammatory, and vulnerary actions.

As an astringent, plantain can help to tighten and tone tissues, particularly those in the digestive system. The most common cause of swollen glands and lymph nodes is an infection in the upper respiratory system; thus, this action may be helpful in reducing excessive mucus secretion in the respiratory system.

As a demulcent, plantain can soothe and moisten irritated or inflamed tissues, particularly those in the respiratory and digestive systems. This action may be helpful in reducing coughs and soothing sore throats.

As an anti-inflammatory, plantain may help reduce swelling and inflammation in the skin and mucous membranes. This action may reduce the symptoms of inflammatory conditions such as eczema and bronchitis.

As a vulnerary, plantain may help promote healing in wounds and injuries, particularly those that are slow to heal or infected. This action may be helpful in reducing the risk of infection and promoting faster healing. Plantain's actions are soothing for raw tissue, and as a remedy it has been known to heal internal wounds that are slow to heal.

Plantain Infusion Recipe:

- Chop 4 tablespoons of fresh plantain leaves (from the narrow leaf or the broad leaf plantains) OR 2 tablespoons of dried plantain leaves and put in a tea ball or tea bag.

- Put in a mug and pour simmering water over the leaves.
- Steep for 5–10 minutes.
- Add honey or maple syrup and lemon (or other aromatic herbs for flavor) if desired.
- For a stronger tea, you can use more plantain.
- Drink 1–2 cups a day as needed.

Plantain Tincture Recipe:

- Chop or grind the plantain leaves and place in a glass jar.
- Pour in enough alcohol to cover, leaving space at the top.*
- Tightly seal the jar, label, date, and shake well.
- Let it steep for 2–3 months. Shake the jar weekly.
- Strain the mixture through cheesecloth.
- Store the tincture in a clean glass jar in a cool place.
- Take 15–20 drops diluted in a small amount of water or juice up to three times a day as needed.
- For children, the proper amount will vary depending on their age and weight. Use 5–7 drops diluted in a small amount of juice or water up to three times a day as needed.

Note: Plantain may be contraindicated for certain medications and may cause side effects such as stomachaches and allergic reactions in some individuals. As with any herbal remedy, it is best to slowly increase the amount used over time and monitor your body's response. Always consult with a clinical herbalist or health care professional before taking herbal remedies, particularly if you have a health-related condition or are taking medication.

Swollen Glands Astringents:

Astringents can help reduce swelling in glands by tightening and toning the tissues. When the tissues are tightened, this helps reduce inflammation and swelling. This is particularly helpful in cases of colds, flu, and other viruses, as these illnesses can cause swollen glands in the neck, armpits, and groin area. Astringents can also help to reduce the production of mucus, thus alleviating congestion and other respiratory symptoms. Some examples of astringent herbs that can be used for swollen glands include echinacea, elderflower, and calendula.

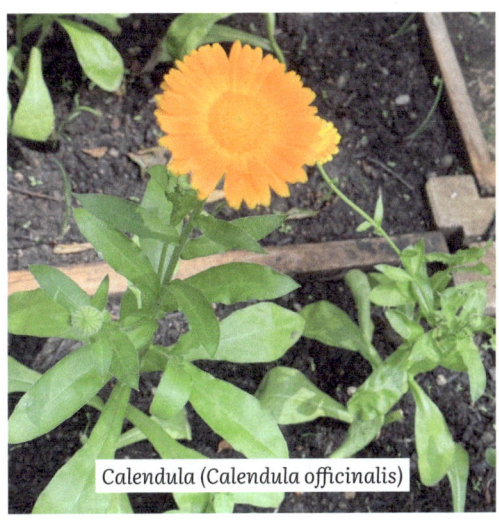
Calendula (Calendula officinalis)

When a person has swollen glands, it often means that the lymphatic system is working to fight off an infection or inflammation in the body. Herbal astringents can be helpful in this process by helping to tighten and tone the tissues in the affected area, reducing inflammation and supporting the body's natural healing process.

Different herbal astringents may have specific actions that make them more effective for swollen glands and the lymph system in various parts of the body. For example, herbal astringents that are particularly helpful for sore throats and swollen tonsils may have a soothing effect on the mucous membranes and tissues in the throat, while astringents that are more beneficial for swollen lymph nodes in the neck may have a more targeted effect on the tissues in that area.

The best choice of herbal astringents will depend on the individual and the specific needs of their body. However, there are several herbs commonly used to support the lymphatic system that may help reduce swollen glands and lymph nodes.

Preparation & Dosage:

A) Cleavers (Galium aparine)
B) Red Clover (Trifolium pratense)
C) Calendula (Calendula officinalis)

D) Yarrow (Achillea millefolium)
E) Elderflower (Sambucus nigra)
F) Echinacea (Purpurea) and echinacea (Angustifolia)
G) Astragalus (Astragalus membranaceus)

Preparation methods for astringent herbs can include teas, tinctures, poultices, and topical applications. It is important to stay hydrated when using astringent herbs, as excessive use can lead to dryness and irritation of the tissues.

Cleavers (Galium aparine)

Cleavers are traditionally used as an astringent for swollen glands due to their ability to reduce inflammation and promote lymphatic drainage. The compounds in cleavers that tighten and tone the lymphatic system and drain swollen glands are tannins called polyphenols.

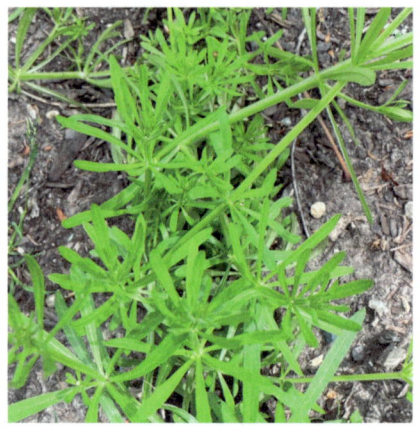

Cleaver Infusion Recipe:

- Place 2–4 teaspoons of fresh cleavers OR 1–2 teaspoons of dried cleavers in a tea ball or tea bag.
- Place in a mug and pour simmering water over the herbs.
- Steep for 10–15 minutes.
- Add honey or maple syrup and lemon if desired.
- Drink an ounce of tea at a time throughout the day. Store in a thermos to keep warm or reheat on the stove. Enjoy 3–4 cups a day as needed until swelling goes down.

Cleavers may take several days or weeks to show effects, so it's important to be patient and consistent with your use.

Note: Cleavers may be contraindicated with certain medications such as blood thinners and diuretics. As with any herbal remedy, it is best to slowly increase the amount used over time and monitor your body's response. Always consult with a clinical herbalist or health care professional before taking herbal remedies, particularly if you have a health-related condition or are taking medication.

Red Clover (Trifolium pratense)

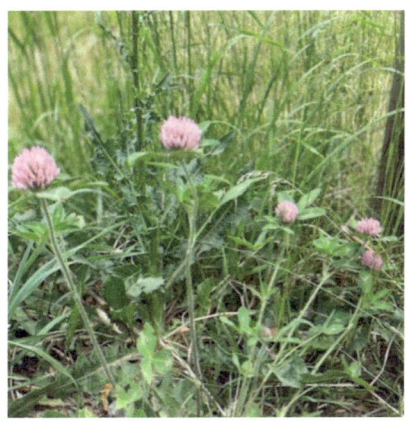

Red clover has traditionally been used as an herbal remedy for swollen glands and other lymphatic conditions when prepared as a tea. Its astringent property comes from isoflavones (compounds that are part of the polyphenol family) and tannins, which tighten, tone, and drain the glands.

Red Clover Infusion Recipe:

- Put 2–3 teaspoons of dried red clover flowers in a tea ball or tea bag.
- Put in a mug and pour simmering water over the herbs.
- Steep for 10–15 minutes.
- Add honey or maple syrup and lemon if desired.
- Drink 1 ounce of tea at a time while it is still warm. Store the rest of the tea in a thermos. Enjoy 1–2 cups a day until the swelling goes down.

Note: Red Clover may take several days or weeks to show its effects, so it's important to be patient and consistent with your use. It is considered a purifier and works on many systems at a time to cleanse toxins out of the body. Always consult with a clinical herbalist or health care professional before taking herbal remedies, particularly if you have a health-related condition or are taking medication.

Calendula (Calendula officinalis)

Calendula is known for its powerful astringent properties, which make it useful for draining swollen glands and lymph nodes. Also, calendula contains carotenoids, they are believed to help protect tissue from oxidative damage caused by free radicals and reduce inflammation and promote wound healing. Carotenoids also heal raw tissue caused by infections internally and externally from wounds. Calendula is packed with tannins that are known to have antimicrobial and anti-inflammatory properties.

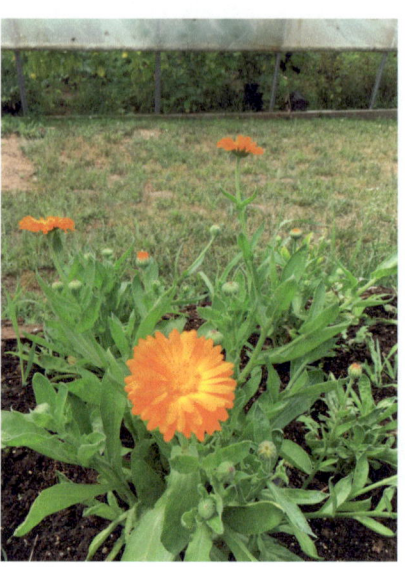

Calendula Infusion Recipe:

Suitable for both internal and topical use.

- Put 1–2 teaspoons of dried calendula flowers in a tea ball or tea bag.
- Place the tea ball or strainer into a mug and pour simmering water over the flowers.
- Steep for 10–15 minutes.
- Add honey or maple syrup and lemon if desired.
- Drink 2–3 cups a day as needed.
- If using topically, let the tea cool down to room temperature, then apply it to the affected area (over the swollen lymph nodes or glands) using a clean cloth or cotton ball.

Calendula can also be used topically as a tincture or infused oil.

Calendula Tincture Recipe:

- Fill a jar with dried calendula flowers.
- Pour in enough alcohol to cover, leaving space at the top.* (For fresh calendula flowers, use Everclear alcohol; it has less water in it to prevent spoilage.)
- Tightly seal the jar, label, date, and shake well.
- Let it steep for 2–3 months. Shake the jar weekly.
- Strain the tincture through cheesecloth and squeeze the liquid out of the herbs.
- Store in a clean glass jar in a dark place.
- Take 10–20 drops diluted with a small amount of water up to three times a day as needed.
- For children, the proper amount will vary depending on their age and weight. Use 5–7 drops diluted in a small amount of juice or water up to three times a day as needed.

Note: As with any herbal remedy, it is best to slowly increase the amount used over time and monitor your body's response. Always consult with a clinical herbalist or health care professional before taking herbal remedies, particularly if you have a health-related condition or are taking medication.

Yarrow (Achillea millefolium)

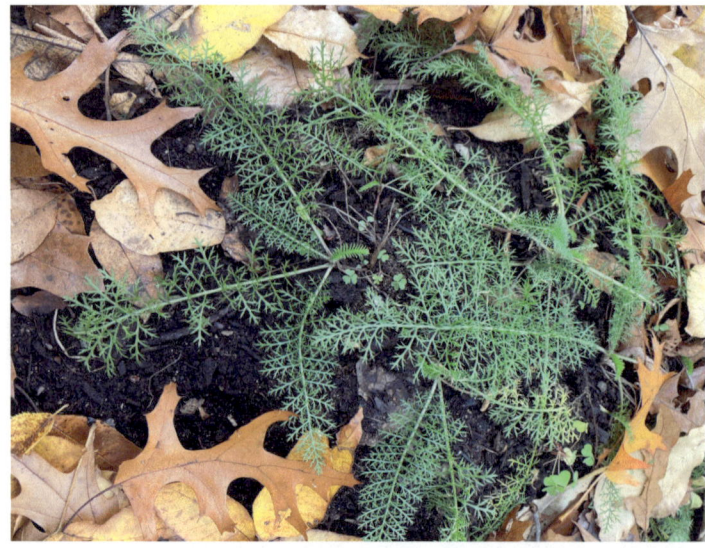

Yarrow contains several compounds with astringent properties, including flavonoids, tannins, and sesquiterpene lactones. These compounds help to tighten and tone tissue, which can be beneficial for swollen glands and lymph nodes.

Yarrow Infusion Recipe:

- Add a handful of fresh yarrow leaves OR 2–4 teaspoons of dried yarrow leaves to a tea ball or tea bag.
- Place into a mug and pour simmering water over the herbs.
- Steep for 5–10 minutes.
- Add honey or maple syrup and lemon if desired.
- Drink 1–3 cups of yarrow tea a day as needed.

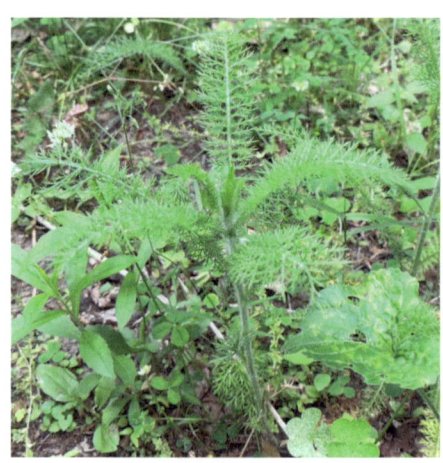

Yarrow Tincture Recipe:

- Fill a jar with fresh or dried yarrow leaves.
- Pour in enough alcohol to cover, leaving space at the top.*
- Tightly seal the jar, label, date, and shake well.
- Let it steep for 2–3 months. Shake the jar weekly.
- Strain and store in a glass jar in a dark place.
- The dosage for yarrow tincture can vary depending on the individual. The standard is to take 15 drops of tincture diluted in water up to three times per day as needed.
- For children, the proper amount will vary depending on their age and weight. Use 5–7 drops diluted in a small amount of juice or water up to three times a day as needed.

Note: Yarrow may cause allergic reactions in some individuals, especially those who are sensitive to plants in the Asteraceae family. It may also be contraindicated with certain medications such as blood thinners and medications metabolized by the liver. Always consult with a clinical herbalist or health care professional before taking herbal remedies, particularly if you have a health-related condition or are taking medication.

Elderflower (Sambucus nigra)

Elderflowers astringent compounds include flavonoids, which are part of the polyphenol family. Their anti-inflammatory actions drain the lymph nodes and swollen glands, while the phenolic acids have antimicrobial and antibacterial properties. Elderflower's powerful oils are antioxidants that protect the raw tissue from viruses or pathogenic organisms.

Elderflower Infusion Recipe:

- Put 2–4 teaspoons of fresh OR dried elderflowers in a tea ball or tea bag.

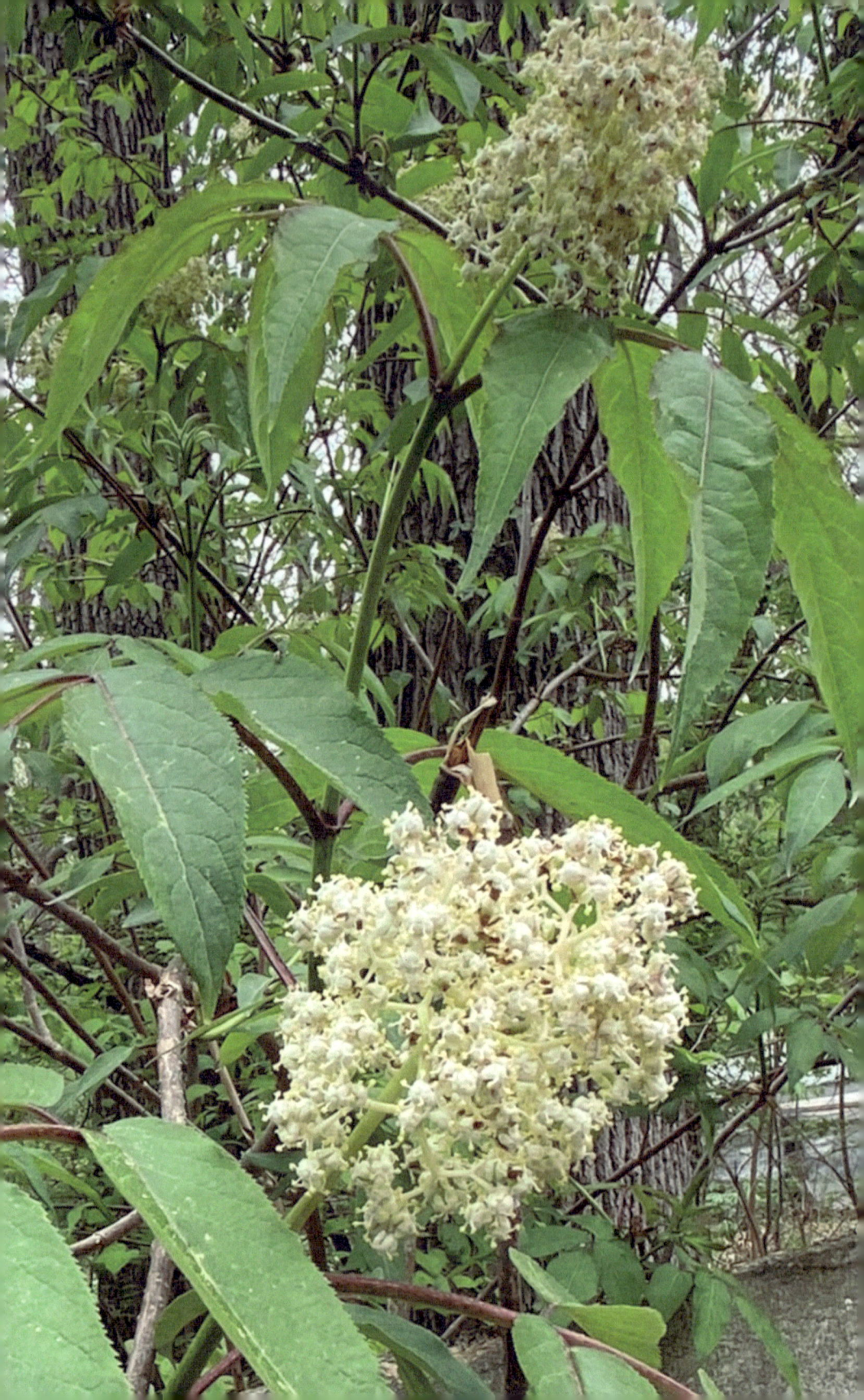

- Place in a mug and pour simmering water over the flowers.
- Steep for 5–10 minutes.
- Add honey or maple syrup and lemon if desired.
- Drink 2–3 cups a day as needed.

Elderflower Tincture Recipe:

- Fill a jar with fresh or dried elder flowers.
- Pour in enough alcohol to cover, leaving space at the top.*
- Tightly seal the jar, label, date, and shake well.
- Let it steep for 2–3 months. Shake the jar weekly.
- Strain and store in a glass jar in a dark place.
- Take 10–20 drops of tincture diluted in water up to three times per day as needed.
- For children, the proper amount will vary depending on their age and weight. Use 5–7 drops diluted in a small amount of juice or water up to three times a day as needed.

Elderflower Syrup Recipe:

- Mix 1 cup of sugar and 1 cup of hot water in a pot. Stir until the sugar dissolves.
- Add 1 cup of dried elderflowers.
- Bring the mixture to a boil, then reduce the heat and simmer for 30 minutes.
- Strain the mixture, return the liquid to the pot, and bring back to a simmer. Stir occasionally until it thickens to a syrup consistency.
- Store the syrup in a clean glass jar in the refrigerator.
- Take 1–2 tablespoons of syrup diluted in water up to three times per day as needed.
- For children, the proper amount will vary depending on their age and weight. Use 1–2 teaspoons diluted in a small amount of juice or water up to three times a day as needed.

Elderflower (Sambucus nigra)

Note: While elderflower is considered safe when used in recommended amounts, always consult with a clinical herbalist or health care professional before taking herbal remedies, particularly if you have a health-related condition or are taking medication.

Echinacea (Purpurea) and Echinacea (Angustifolia)

Both echinacea purpurea and echinacea angustifolia have been used as astringents for swollen glands and lymph nodes. They have traditionally been used for their astringent and anti-inflammatory properties to help reduce swelling and inflammation in the lymphatic system, especially when treating colds, flus, viruses, and other respiratory infections.

Echinacea Topical Compress:

- Add water and echinacea root to a pot.
- Bring to a boil and let the mixture boil for 5 minutes.
- Remove from heat and steep for 15 minutes.
- Strain the mixture.
- Soak a cotton cloth in the hot infusion and wring out the excess.
- Apply the hot cloth to the affected area. Let it sit for 10–15 minutes.
- Repeat the process throughout the day for relief as needed.

Echinacea Flower Infusion Recipe:

- Put 1 tablespoon of dried echinacea flowers in a tea ball or tea bag.
- Place in a mug and pour boiling water over the flowers.
- Steep for 5–10 minutes.
- Add honey or maple syrup and lemon if desired.
- Enjoy up to four times a day as needed (or twice a day for children).

Echinacea Root Decoction Recipe:

- Put 1 tablespoon of chopped dried echinacea root in a pot with 2 cups of water.
- Bring to a boil, then reduce the heat and let it simmer for 15–20 minutes.
- Strain the tea into a mug.
- Add honey or maple syrup and lemon if desired.
- Enjoy up to two times a day as needed (or once a day for children).

Echinacea Tincture Recipe:

- Fill a clean glass jar about ⅔ full of dried echinacea.
- Pour in enough alcohol to cover, leaving space at the top.*
- Tightly seal the jar, label, date, and shake well.
- Let it steep for 2–3 months. Shake the jar weekly.
- Strain the tincture through cheesecloth into a clean glass jar. Squeeze the cheesecloth to extract all the liquid from the herbs.
- Store in a jar in a dark place.
- Take 10–20 drops diluted with a little bit of water up to three times a day as needed.
- For children, the proper amount will vary depending on their age and weight. Use 3–5 drops diluted in a small amount of juice or water up to three times a day as needed.

Note: Do not consume echinacea for extended periods of time (no more than 8 weeks), as overuse may negatively affect the liver and immune system. Always consult with a clinical herbalist or health care professional before taking herbal remedies, particularly if you have a health-related condition or are taking medication.

Astringent Food & Recipes

Foods with Astringent Actions

- Blackberries, blueberries, and raspberries all contain high levels of tannins, which have astringent properties.
- Pomegranate juice contains tannins and other compounds that have been shown to have astringent properties.
- Green tea contains a compound called epigallocatechin gallate (EGCG) that has been shown to have astringent properties.
- Apples contain a type of soluble fiber called pectin that has been shown to have astringent properties.
- Beans and legumes contain soluble fiber and other compounds that have been shown to have astringent properties.
- Cruciferous vegetables, broccoli, cabbage, and Brussels sprouts all contain compounds called glycosylates that have astringent properties.
- Quince is a fruit that is high in tannins and has been traditionally used for its astringent properties.

Recipes with Astringent Properties

Apple Cider Vinegar Tonic:

- 2 tablespoons apple cider vinegar
- 1 tablespoon honey
- 1 cup water
- Mix all ingredients together as a tonic daily.

Apple cider vinegar is a natural astringent that can help regulate the body's pH balance.

Berry Smoothie:

- 1 cup frozen mixed berries, raspberries, and blackberries OR berries of your choice

- ½ banana
- ½ cup non-dairy yogurt
- ½ cup unsweetened almond milk
- 1 tablespoon chia seeds
- Blend all ingredients together until smooth.

Berries contain tannins, natural astringents that can help tighten and tone tissues.

Quinoa Salad:

- 2 cups cooked quinoa
- ½ cup cooked garbanzo beans
- ½ cup cubed cucumber
- ⅓ cup cubed tomato
- ¼ cup diced red onion
- ¼ cup chopped fresh parsley
- 2 tablespoons extra virgin olive oil
- 1 tablespoon of lemon juice
- Salt and pepper
- Mix all ingredients together and enjoy.

Quinoa is a good source for tannins that have natural astringent effects.

Green Tea:

- 1 bag of green tea
- 1 cup simmering water
- Steep the green tea bag in the boiling water for 3–5 minutes.

Green tea contains tannins that have natural astringent properties.

Note: It is important to note that while these foods and drinks do possess astringent properties, they should not be relied upon as a sole treatment for any condition.

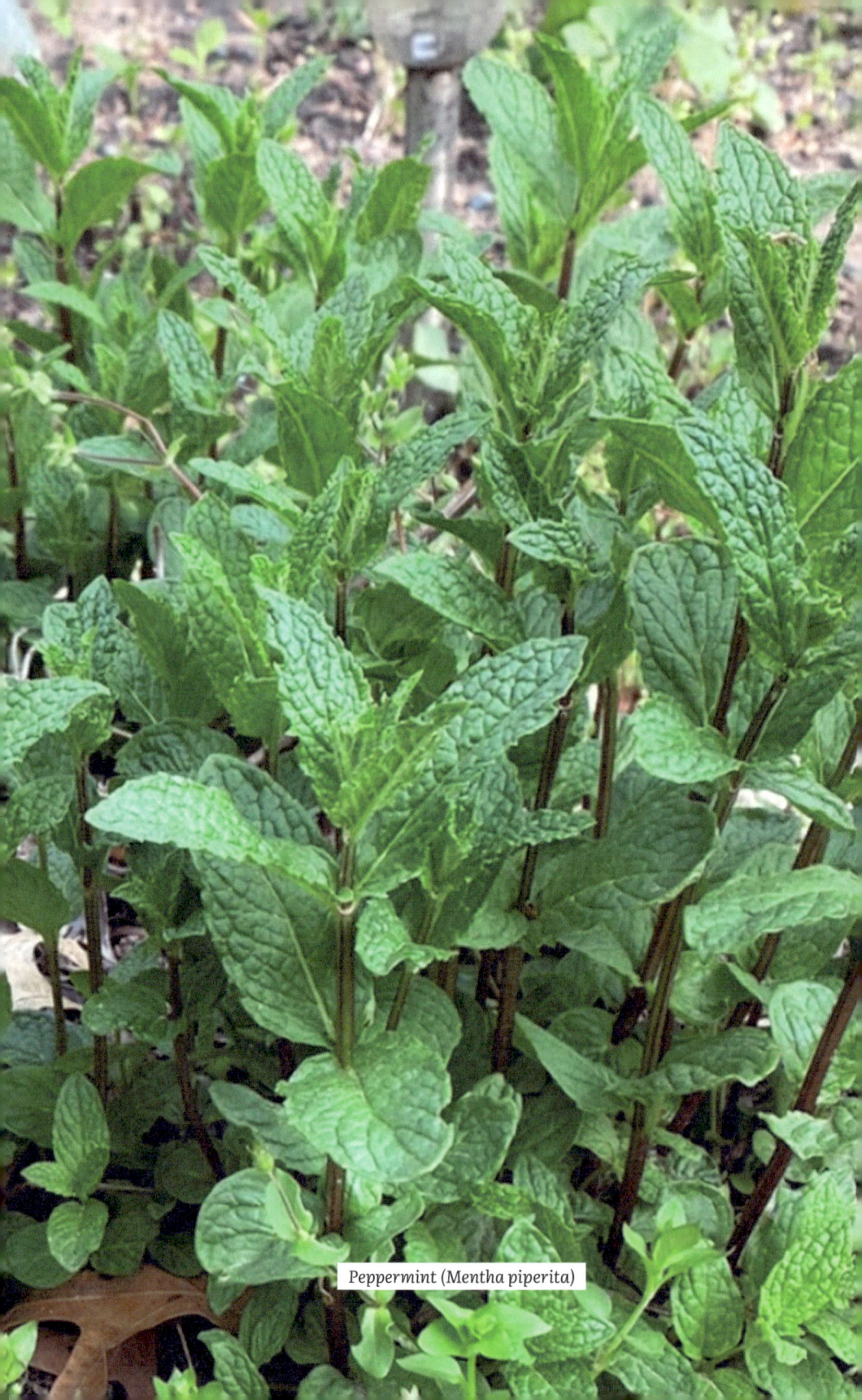
Peppermint (Mentha piperita)

CHAPTER 6.
CARMINATIVE HERBS

Carminative herbs help soothe the digestive system by reducing gas and bloating, easing cramping, and restoring the health of the intestinal wall.

- A) Fennel (Foeniculum vulgare)
- B) Ginger (Zingiber officinale)
- C) Cumin (Cuminum cyminum)
- D) Anise (Pimpinella anisum)
- E) Chamomile (Matricaria chamomilla)
- F) Licorice (Glycyrrhiza glabra)
- G) Peppermint (Mentha piperita)

Preparation & Dosage

Fennel (Foeniculum vulgare)

Fennel contains several volatile oils (including anethole, fenchone, and estragole) that have carminative properties. These compounds can help relax the smooth muscles of the digestive tract, reducing spasms and cramping. Fennel can also stimulate the production of digestive enzymes, aiding in the digestion of food and helping to prevent indigestion. Additionally, fennel's anti-inflammatory properties may reduce inflammation in the digestive tract and soothe both bloating and gas. These actions make fennel an effective carminative herb to relieve digestive discomfort and promote healthy digestion.

Fennel Infusion Recipe:

- Add 1–2 teaspoons of crushed fennel seeds to a tea ball.
- Place in a mug and pour simmering water over the herbs.
- Steep for 5–10 minutes.
- Add honey or other herbs for flavor if desired.
- For a stronger infusion, add more fennel seeds.
- Drink up to three times a day after meals.

Fennel Essential Oil:

Fennel essential oil can also be used as a carminative.

- Dilute the essential oil by blending 1–2 drops of fennel essential oil with a teaspoon of carrier oil. (Use 10 drops to an ounce of oil.)
- Rub over the abdomen and gallbladder area to the right of the rib cage.

Note: Fennel may be contraindicated with certain medications, including blood thinners and some medications for seizures. Fennel should also be avoided or used with caution in people with allergies to plants in the carrot family. As with any herbal remedy, it is best to slowly increase the amount used over time and monitor your body's response. Always consult with a clinical herbalist or health care professional before taking herbal remedies, particularly if you have a health-related condition or are taking medication.

Ginger (Zingiber officinale)

Ginger contains several active compounds such as gingerols and shogaols that give it its carminative properties. These compounds can help to relax the smooth muscles of the digestive tract, thus reducing spasms and cramping. Ginger can also stimulate the production of digestive enzymes and aid in the digestion of food and prevent indigestion. Ginger's anti-inflammatory actions may also reduce inflammation in the digestive tract and soothe bloating and gas.

Ginger Infusion Recipe:

- Add 1–2 teaspoons of sliced fresh ginger OR ½–1 teaspoons of grated dried ginger to a tea bag or tea ball.
- Place in a mug and pour boiling water over the ginger.
- Steep for 5–10 minutes.
- Add honey or maple syrup and lemon if desired.
- For a stronger tea, you can use more ginger root.
- Drink 1–3 mugs of ginger tea a day as needed.

Ginger Capsules:

- Ginger capsules are also available commercially. Be sure to follow the instructions on the product label or as directed by a clinical herbalist or a health care provider.
- Capsules typically contain dried ginger root extract and may be standardized to a certain concentration of gingerols and shogaols.

Note: Ginger may be contraindicated with certain medications such as blood thinners and some medications for diabetes and high blood pressure. Ginger may also cause side effects such as heartburn, nausea, and allergic reactions in some individuals. As with any herbal remedy, it is best to slowly increase the amount used over time and monitor your body's response. Always consult with a clinical herbalist or health care professional before taking herbal remedies, particularly if you have a health-related condition or are taking medication.

Cumin (Cuminum cyminum)

Cumin seeds contain essential oils such as cuminaldehyde and thymol that possess anti-inflammatory and anti-spasmodic effects. These compounds help to relax the smooth muscles in the digestive tract and reduce inflammation, which helps alleviate symptoms of bloating, gas, and cramping. Additionally, cumin can stimulate the production of digestive enzymes and aid in the breakdown of food and promote healthy digestion. These actions make cumin an effective carminative herb capable of relieving digestive discomfort and promoting healthy digestion.

Black cumin seeds can be prepared as an oil infusion either for ingestion or topical use to obtain its carminative benefits. You can also grind them in a mortar and pestle and add the powder to your soups, stir-fries, or casseroles.

Powdered Black Cumin Seeds Recipe:

Ingredients:

- ¼ cup black cumin seeds
- 1 cup oil (such as olive oil, coconut oil, or sesame oil)

Preparation:

- Place the black cumin seeds in a mortar and pestle and gently crush them to release their oils. You can also use a coffee grinder or food processor.
- In a small saucepan, heat the oil over low heat until it is hot but not boiling.
- Add the crushed black cumin seeds to the hot oil and stir to combine. Turn off the heat.
- Steep anywhere from 1 hour up to 10 days in a warm place away from direct sunlight.
- Strain the oil using cheesecloth and store the oil in a glass jar or bottle in the refrigerator.
- Take 1 teaspoon of cumin oil before a meal for its carminative effects.

Note: You can also use this topically to relieve muscle pain and inflammation.

Cumin Infusion Recipe:

- Add 1–2 teaspoons of ground cumin seeds in a tea bag.
- Place in a mug and pour simmering water over the seeds.
- Steep for 5 minutes.
- Add honey or maple syrup and lemon (or other aromatic herbs for flavor) if desired.
- For a stronger tea, you can use more cumin seeds.
- Drink 1–3 cups a day, preferably after meals.

Cumin Essential Oil:

Cumin essential oil can also be used as a carminative, but it should be diluted with an oil as it could be irritating to the skin.

- Dilute the essential oil by blending 1–2 drops of cumin essential oil with a teaspoon of carrier oil. (Use 10 drops to an ounce of oil.)
- Rub over the abdomen, up the ribs on the right side, and over the gallbladder.

Note: Cumin may be contraindicated with certain medications such as blood thinners and medications for diabetes and high blood pressure. Cumin should also be used with caution in individuals with allergies to plants in the parsley family. As with any herbal remedy, it is best to slowly increase the amount used over time and monitor your body's response. Always consult with a clinical herbalist or health care professional before taking herbal remedies, particularly if you have a health-related condition or are taking medication.

Anise (Pimpinella anisum)

Anise contains volatile oils such as anethole with carminative properties that may relax the muscles in the digestive tract, reducing spasms and cramping. This helps to relieve gas and bloating and promotes healthy digestion. Anise also has antimicrobial properties that can reduce the growth of bad bacteria in the gut that may contribute to digestive issues. Anise as a carminative is effective for relieving gas, cramps, and nausea.

Anise Infusion Recipe:

- Add 1–2 teaspoons of crushed anise seeds to a tea ball or tea bag.
- Place in a mug and pour simmering water over the seeds.
- Steep for 5–10 minutes.
- Drink 1–3 cups per day as needed.

Anise Capsules:

- Anise capsules are available commercially. Follow the dosage instructions on the product label.

Anise Aromatherapy:

- Use 2–3 drops of anise essential oil in a diffuser.
- Alternatively, sprinkle 2–3 drops of anise essential oil on a paper towel or cotton ball and inhale directly for a few minutes.

Anise Tincture Recipe:

- Crush 1 cup of anise seeds in a mortar and pestle or grind them in a coffee grinder.
- Place the anise seeds in a clean glass jar.
- Pour in enough alcohol to cover, leaving space at the top.*
- Tightly seal the jar, label, date, and shake well.
- Let it steep for 2–3 months. Shake the jar weekly.

- Strain the mixture through cheesecloth into a clean jar.
- Store the tincture in a dark place.
- Take 7–10 drops of the tincture diluted in a small amount of water up to three times a day as needed.
- For children, the proper amount will vary depending on their age and weight. Use 3–5 drops diluted in a small amount of juice or water up to three times a day as needed.

Note: Use anise in moderation to avoid unwanted side effects. Anise may be contraindicated with certain medications. Always consult with a clinical herbalist or health care professional before taking herbal remedies, particularly if you have a health-related condition or are taking medication.

Chamomile (Matricaria chamomilla)

Chamomile contains essential oils (primarily alpha-bisabolol and chamazulene) with carminative properties. These compounds help to relax smooth muscles, reduce spasms, and cramping in the digestive tract. With its anti-inflammatory properties, chamomile may also help reduce inflammation in the digestive system. Chamomile has been used as both a tea and a tincture for its carminative properties to soothe digestive discomfort, bloating, gas, and indigestion.

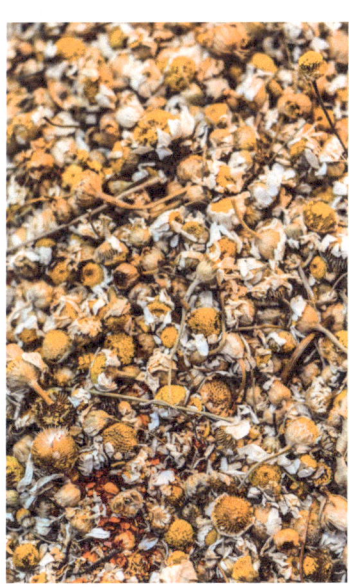

Chamomile Infusion Recipe:

- Put 2 teaspoons of dried chamomile flowers in a tea bag or tea ball.
- Place in a mug and pour simmering water over the flowers.

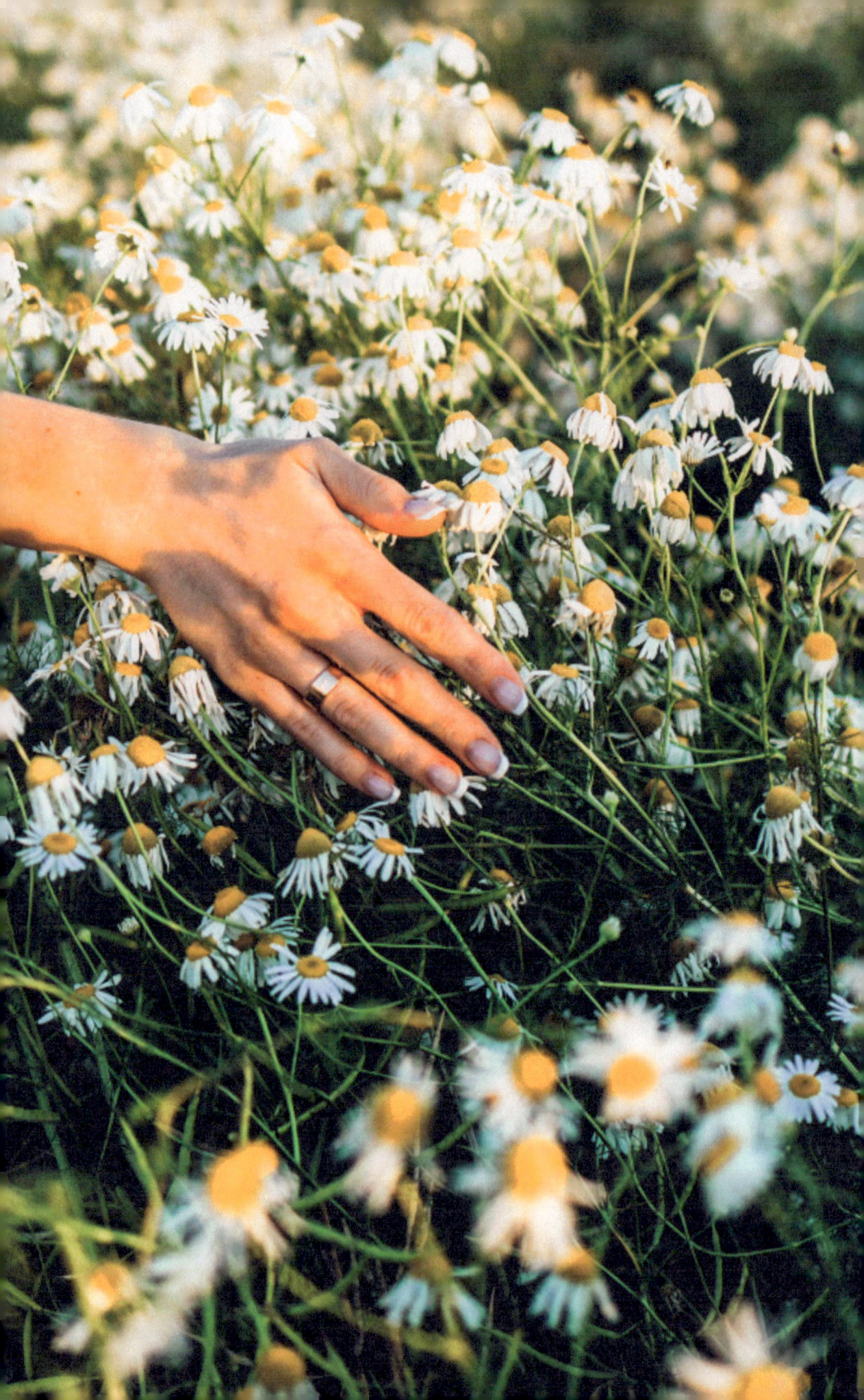

- Steep for 5 minutes.
- Add honey or maple syrup and lemon if desired.
- Drink 1–3 mugs per day as needed.

Chamomile Tincture Recipe:

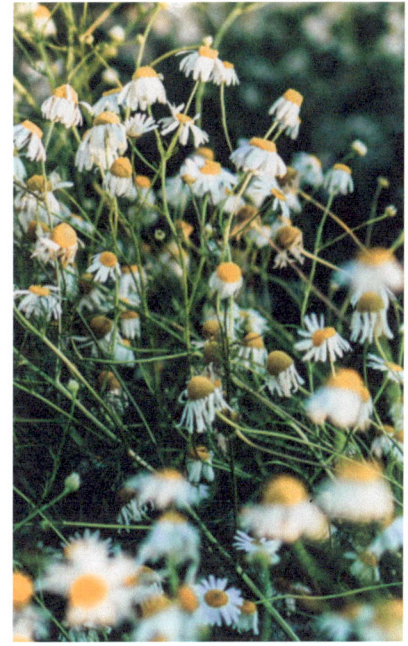

- Put dried chamomile flowers in a glass jar.
- Pour in enough alcohol to cover, leaving space at the top.*
- Tightly seal the jar, label, date, and shake well.
- Let it steep for 2–3 months. Shake the jar weekly.
- Strain the mixture through cheese cloth and squeeze the cloth to release the remainder of the liquid.
- Store the tincture in a clean jar in a dark place.
- Take 10–15 drops diluted in a little bit of water up to three times per day as needed.
- For children, the proper amount will vary depending on their age and weight. Use 3–5 drops diluted in a small amount of juice or water up to three times a day as needed.

Note: While chamomile is considered safe for most people, it can cause allergic reactions in some individuals, particularly those with allergies to plants in the daisy family. It may also be contraindicated with certain medications. Always consult with a clinical herbalist or health care professional before taking herbal remedies, particularly if you have a health-related condition or are taking medication.

Chamomile (Matricaria chamomilla)

Licorice (Glycyrrhiza glabra)

Licorice contains saponins and flavonoid compounds that have been shown to have antispasmodic properties, making it an effective carminative. These compounds relax the muscles in the digestive tract, reducing cramping and discomfort. Licorice also contains glycyrrhizin, a sweet-tasting compound that has been shown to stimulate the production of mucus in the stomach lining, helping to protect it from damage caused by excess acid.

In addition to its carminative properties, licorice has been traditionally used for its anti-inflammatory and demulcent properties that aid in soothing and protecting the lining of the digestive tract. This makes licorice a useful herb for heartburn, indigestion, and ulcers.

Licorice Infusion Recipe:

- Chop 1–2 teaspoons of dried licorice root and add to a pot with 2 cups of water.
- Bring to a boil and let it boil for 5 minutes.
- Remove from heat and steep for 5 minutes.
- Drink up to three cups per day as needed.

Licorice Tincture Recipe:

- Fill a glass jar with 1 cup of dried licorice root.
- Pour in enough alcohol to cover, leaving space at the top.*
- Tightly seal the jar, label, date, and shake well.
- Let it steep for 2–3 months. Shake the jar weekly.
- Strain the liquid through cheese cloth and discard the solids.
- Transfer the liquid to a glass jar.
- Take 5–7 drops diluted in a little bit of water up to three times a day as needed.
- For children, the proper amount will vary depending on their age and weight. Use 3–5 drops diluted in a small amount of juice or water up to two times a day as needed.

Note: While licorice can be an effective carminative, it can also have side effects in some individuals. Licorice contains glycyrrhizin, which, when consumed in large amounts or over long periods of time, can lead to high blood pressure and low potassium levels. Licorice should also not be used by people with high blood pressure, as it can raise blood pressure levels in some individuals. Always consult with a clinical herbalist or health care professional before taking herbal remedies, particularly if you have a health-related condition or are taking medication.

Peppermint (Mentha piperita)

Peppermint contains compounds such as menthol and terpenes that have a relaxing effect on the digestive tract, helping to reduce spasms and cramps. It also stimulates the flow of bile and digestive juices, aiding in the digestion of fats and the relief of bloating and gas. These actions make peppermint an effective carminative that promotes healthy digestion.

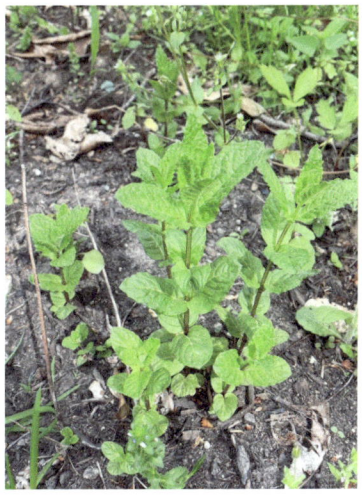

Peppermint Infusion Recipe:

- Add 2–4 teaspoons of chopped fresh peppermint leaves OR 2 teaspoons of dried peppermint leaves to a tea ball or tea bag.
- Place into a mug and pour simmering water over the herbs.
- Steep for 5–10 minutes.
- Add honey or maple syrup and lemon (or other aromatic herbs for flavor) if desired.
- For a stronger tea, you can use more peppermint leaves.
- Drink up to three cups a day after meals.

Peppermint essential oil can be used in several ways, but it's important to note that essential oils are highly concentrated and should be used with caution. Here are some common preparations and dosages for peppermint essential oil:

Peppermint Steam Vapor:

- Sprinkle a few drops of peppermint essential oil into a bowl of simmering water.

Cover your head and the bowl with a towel and inhale the steam for several minutes.

- Alternatively, sprinkle a few drops into a diffuser or humidifier and breathe in the aroma. Inhalation of peppermint oil can help relieve congestion and promote mental clarity.

Topical Application:

- Peppermint essential oil can be diluted with a carrier oil (such as virgin coconut oil, olive oil, or jojoba oil) and applied to the skin over the abdomen for pain relief or relaxation.
- Mix 1-2 drops of peppermint oil with 1 teaspoon of carrier oil or 10 drops to an ounce of carrier oil and massage into the skin.
- Avoid applying peppermint oil to sensitive areas or broken skin.

Note: Peppermint should not be taken in large amounts or for extended periods of time, as it can lead to heartburn, ulcers, nausea, and allergic reactions. Peppermint should also be avoided or used with caution in individuals with gastroesophageal reflux disease (GERD), as it can exacerbate symptoms. As with any herbal remedy, it is best to slowly increase the amount used over time and monitor your body's response. Always consult with a clinical herbalist or health care professional before taking herbal remedies, particularly if you have a health-related condition or are taking medication.

Carminative Foods and Recipes

- Ginger tea, ginger chews, or fresh ginger added to meals.
- Roasted fennel, fennel tea, or fennel seeds are added to meals.
- Peppermint tea or fresh peppermint added to meals.
- Chamomile tea or fresh chamomile added to meals.
- Cumin oil and crushed cumin seeds are added to meals or ground cumin as a spice in cooking.
- Coriander seeds are added to meals or as a spice in cooking.
- Dill seeds or fresh dill added to meals or as a garnish.
- Cardamom pods or ground cardamom added to meals or as a spice in cooking.

Some recipes that incorporate these carminative foods and herbs include:

Ginger Tea:

- Boil water and add slices of fresh ginger.
- Add fresh lemon and honey to taste.

Roasted Fennel Salad:

- Slice fennel bulbs and roast them with olive oil and salt.
- Toss with arugula, lemon juice, and shaved parmesan.

Peppermint and Chamomile Tea:

- Steep peppermint and chamomile tea bags in hot water for 5–10 minutes
- Add honey or maple syrup and lemon to taste.

Cumin and Coriander Roasted Carrots:

- Toss baby carrots with olive oil.

- Add ground cumin and coriander, then roast in the oven until tender.

Dill Yogurt Dip:

- Mix plain yogurt, chopped fresh dill, lemon juice, and salt together.
- Eat as a dip with vegetables or pita chips for a snack or appetizer.

Cardamom Spiced Oatmeal:

- Cook oat groats or oat flakes.
- Add ground cardamom, chopped nuts, and honey to warm oatmeal for a soothing breakfast.

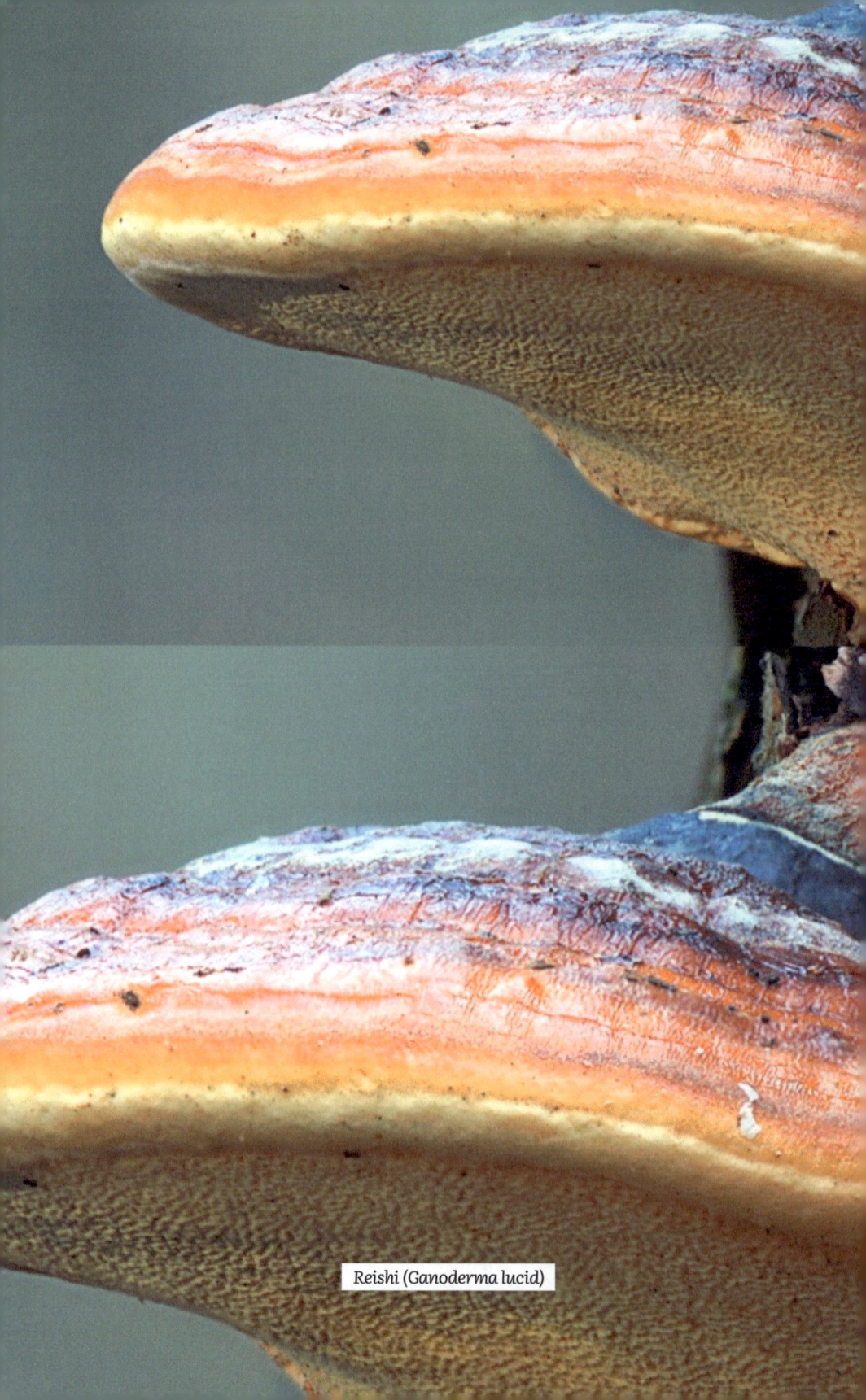

Reishi (Ganoderma lucid)

CHAPTER 7.
ADAPTOGEN HERBS

Rejuvenating herbs restore vitality and energy to the body after a stressful infection as well as promote overall health and well-being. Some rejuvenating herbs boost the immune system's function. Astragalus and ashwagandha are two examples of adaptogenic herbs with immune-boosting properties that help to enhance the body's natural defenses against infections and illnesses by restoring the body's homeostasis. Reishi and ginseng, on the other hand, protect the body from the lingering effects of stress that may cause low energy and chronic disease.

A) Ashwagandha (Withania somnifera)
B) Astragalus (Astragalus membranaceus)
C) Ginseng (Panax ginseng)
D) Reishi (Ganoderma lucidum)
E) Eleuthero (Eleutherococctus senticosus)

Preparation methods for rejuvenating herbs can include teas, tinctures, capsules, and powdered extracts.

Preparation & Dosage

Ashwagandha (Withania somnifera)[3]

Ashwagandha supports immune function by enhancing antibody production, reducing inflammation, boosting antioxidant activity, reducing stress, and increasing white blood cell count. Some preliminary studies suggest that ashwagandha may have antiviral properties as well and could potentially be useful in treating viral infections.

The herbal medicine *Withania somnifera* has an excellent antiviral activity that could be implicated in the management and treatment of flu and flu-like diseases connected with SARS-CoV-2 (Covid-19).

At present, synthetic adjuvant vaccines are used against COVID-19. Available information showed the antiviral activity in Withanoside V of *Withania somnifera*, which may explore as herbal medicine against to SARS-CoV-2 infection after standardization of parameters of drug development and formulation in near future.

Ashwagandha Powder:

- Grind dried Ashwagandha root into powder.
- This powder can be mixed with warm water, milk, or honey to make a tonic.
- Take 1–2 teaspoons up to three times per day as needed.
- It can be taken on an empty stomach.

Ashwagandha Capsules:

---

[3] Singh, M., Jayant, K., Singh, D., Bhutani, S., Poddar, N. K., Chaudhary, A. A., Khan, S. U. D., Adnan, M., Siddiqui, A. J., Hassan, M. I., Khan, F. I., Lai, D., & Khan, S. (2022, July 11). *Withania somnifera* (L.) Dunal (Ashwagandha) for the possible therapeutics and clinical management of SARS-CoV-2 infection: Plant-based drug discovery and targeted therapy. Frontiers. https://doi.org/10.3389/fcimb.2022.933824

- Ashwagandha is also available commercially in capsule form. These can be taken orally with water.

Ashwagandha Decoction Recipe:

- Chop 1 tablespoon of fresh Ashwagandha root OR 1 teaspoon of dried Ashwagandha root.
- Bring 2 cups of water to a boil in a small saucepan.
- Add chopped Ashwagandha root.
- Reduce heat and let the mixture simmer for 15 minutes.
- Strain the tea into a mug.
- Add honey or maple syrup and lemon for flavor if desired.
- Drink 1–2 cups per day as needed.

Ashwagandha Tincture Recipe:

- Chop 1 cup of dried ashwagandha root and place in a clean glass jar.
- Pour in enough alcohol to cover, leaving space at the top.*
- Tightly seal the jar, label, date, and shake well.
- Let it steep for 2–3 months. Shake the jar weekly.
- Strain the mixture, then store it in a glass jar in a dark place.
- Take 10–15 drops diluted in a small amount of water or juice up to three times per day.
- For children, the proper amount will vary depending on their age and weight. Use 5–7 drops diluted in a small amount of juice or water up to three times a day as needed.

Note: Excessive use of Ashwagandha tincture can lead to unwanted side effects. Ashwagandha may also be contraindicated with certain medications. Always consult with a clinical herbalist or health care professional before taking herbal remedies, particularly if you have a health-related condition or are taking medication.

Astragalus (Astragalus membranaceus)

Astragalus is a traditional Chinese herb that has been used for centuries for its immune-boosting properties. It has been shown to be essential for fighting off infections and illnesses.

Astragalus has been found to enhance the production of antibodies, possess strong anti-inflammatory properties, and stimulate interferon production, the proteins vital in boosting the immune response to fight off viral infections. Its antioxidant compounds also help to protect the body's cells from the damage free radicals can cause, thus supporting immune function and overall health.

Astragalus Decoction Recipe:

- Add 1–2 teaspoons of dried astragalus root to a pot of water and bring to a boil.
- Reduce heat and simmer for 20 minutes.
- Strain the mixture.
- Drink 2–3 mugs a day as needed.

Astragalus Tincture Recipe:

- Fill a jar ⅔ full with dried astragalus root.
- Pour in enough alcohol to cover, leaving space at the top.*
- Tightly seal the jar, label, date, and shake well.
- Let it steep for 2–3 months. Shake the jar weekly.
- Strain the mixture, then store it in a glass jar in a dark place.
- Take 7–10 drops of tincture diluted in a small amount of water up to three times per day as needed.
- For children, the proper amount will vary depending on their age and weight. Use 3–5 drops diluted in a small amount of juice or water up to three times a day as needed.

Astragalus Capsules:

- Astragalus is also available commercially in capsule form. These can be taken orally with water.

Note: Excessive use of astragalus can lead to unwanted side effects. It may also be contraindicated with certain medications. Always consult with a clinical herbalist or health care professional before taking herbal remedies, particularly if you have a health-related condition or are taking medication.

Ginseng (Panax ginseng)

Ginseng is another herb historically used in TCM that has been used for centuries for its rejuvenating properties. It supports overall health and well-being by increasing energy levels, combating fatigue, enhancing physical endurance and mental focus, reducing chronic stress, and boosting overall mood. With these properties, ginseng is a popular supplement among athletes and students.

Ginseng regulates the body's immune response and hormonal changes due to stress and stimulates the immune system, helping to maintain homeostasis and protect against infections and illnesses.

Ginseng has also been known to be an aphrodisiac and is referred to as a "male herb."

In addition, ginseng has been shown to improve cognitive function, memory, attention span, and processing speed.

Ginseng Decoction Recipe:

- Add 2 teaspoons of dried ginseng root to a mug.
- Pour simmering water over the ginseng and cover the mug.
- Simmer for 10–15 minutes, then strain.

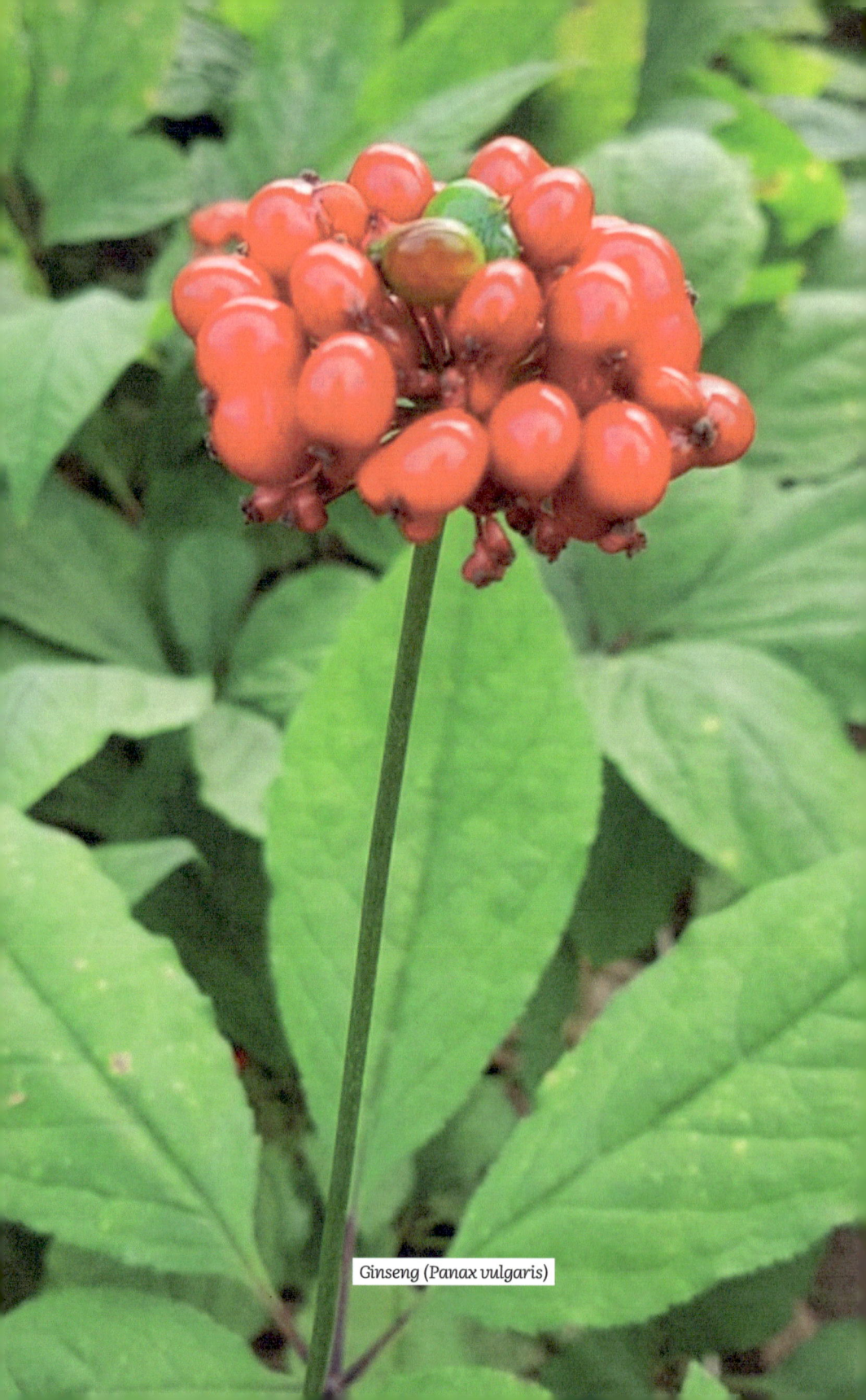
Ginseng (Panax vulgaris)

- You can save the roots and reuse them for another mug of tea.
- Sweeten with honey or maple syrup and lemon if desired.
- Drink 1–2 cups of ginseng tea per day. However, it is a stimulant; drink it earlier in the day to ensure a good night's sleep.

Ginseng Tincture Recipe:

- Crush or chop ginseng root into small pieces and place in a jar.
- Pour in enough alcohol to cover, leaving space at the top.*
- Tightly seal the jar, label, date, and shake well.
- Let it steep for 2–3 months. Shake the jar weekly.
- Strain the mixture, then store it in a glass jar in a dark place.
- Take 10 drops of tincture diluted in a small amount of water up to three times per day.
- Ginseng tincture is not recommended for children.

Ginseng Capsules:

- Ginseng is also available in capsule form commercially. Follow the directions for usage on the label.

Note: Long-term use or large amounts of ginseng may lead to headaches, dizziness, stomach upset, and other adverse symptoms. Always consult with a clinical herbalist or health care professional before taking herbal remedies, particularly if you have a health-related condition or are taking medication.

Reishi (Ganoderma lucidum)

Reishi has long been used in TCM for its rejuvenating properties. Reishi supports overall health and well-being by activating the immune system, reducing chronic inflammation, protecting the body's cells with its antioxidant properties, and producing a calming effect on the body that can result in reduced stress, increased relaxation, and improved sleep quality.

Reishi Decoction Recipe:

- Bring 2 cups of water to a boil.
- Add 2 teaspoons of dried reishi mushroom.
- Reduce heat and simmer for 20–30 minutes with the lid on.
- Strain the mixture and save the reishi for another decoction.
- Add honey or maple syrup and lemon to the tea if desired.
- Drink 1–2 cups of reishi decoction per day as needed.

Reishi Tincture Recipe:

- Place dried reishi mushroom in a jar.
- Pour in enough alcohol to cover, leaving space at the top.*
- Tightly seal the jar, label, date, and shake well.
- Let it steep for 2–3 months. Shake the jar weekly.
- Strain the mixture, then store it in a glass jar in a dark place.
- Take 10–15 drops of tincture diluted in a small amount of water up to three times per day as needed.
- For children, the proper amount will vary depending on their age and weight. Use 5–7 drops diluted in a small amount of juice or water up to three times a day as needed.

Reishi Capsules:

- Reishi is also available commercially in capsule form. Follow the directions for usage on the label.

Note: Excessive use of reishi can lead to unwanted side effects. It may also be contraindicated with certain medications. Always consult with a clinical herbalist or health care professional before taking herbal remedies, particularly if you have a health-related condition or are taking medication.

Eleuthero (Eleutherococcus senticosus)

Eleuthero, also called Siberian ginseng, is an adaptogenic herb that helps the body adapt to stress and maintain a balanced homeostasis. This is crucial when recovering from an illness, and utilizing rejuvenating herbs during illness results in a quicker overall recovery.

Adaptogens like eleuthero have been found to support the body's natural stress response system, helping to regulate stress hormones and promote a sense of calm and balance. This can help improve overall health and well-being.

In addition to its rejuvenating and adaptogenic actions, eleuthero has also been found to support the immune system, protect against infections, and exhibit antioxidant properties that break down free radicals that cause oxidative stress and damage to the body's cells.

Eleuthero Decoction Recipe:

- Chop 2 tablespoons of dried eleuthero root and add to a pot with a quart of water.
- Bring to a boil, then reduce the heat and simmer for 20–30 minutes.
- Strain the mixture.
- Add honey or maple syrup and lemon to the tea, if desired.
- Drink 1–2 cups as needed. However, drink this earlier in the day, as eleuthero is a stimulant.

Eleuthero Tincture Recipe:

- Place dried eleuthero root in a glass jar.
- Pour in enough alcohol to cover, leaving space at the top.*
- Tightly seal the jar, label, date, and shake well.
- Let it steep for 2–3 months. Shake the jar weekly.
- Strain the mixture, then store it in a glass jar in a dark place.

- Take 7–10 drops of tincture diluted in a small amount of water up to three times per day as needed.
- For children, the proper amount will vary depending on their age and weight. Use 3–5 drops diluted in a small amount of juice or water up to three times a day as needed.

Eleuthero Capsules:

- Eleuthero is also available commercially in capsule form. Follow the instructions for usage on the label.

Note: Excessive use of eleuthero can lead to unwanted side effects. It may also be contraindicated with certain medications. Always consult with a clinical herbalist or health care professional before taking herbal remedies, particularly if you have a health-related condition or are taking medication.

Rejuvenating Adaptogen Foods and Recipes

Ashwagandha Latte:

Ingredients:

- 1 cup milk or nondairy milk (almond, coconut, etc.)
- 1 tsp ashwagandha powder
- 1 tsp natural sweetener, such as honey or maple syrup (optional)
- ½ tsp cinnamon (optional)

Instructions:

- Heat the milk until it is warm.
- Add ashwagandha powder and sweetener (if using) and whisk until blended.
- Add cinnamon (if using), pour into your favorite mug, and enjoy.

Turmeric Ginger Tea:

Ingredients:

- 2 cups water
- 1-inch piece sliced fresh ginger
- 1-inch piece sliced fresh turmeric
- 1 tbsp honey or maple syrup
- Juice of ½ lemon

Instructions:

- Heat water until it is simmering.
- Add ginger and turmeric. Cover the pot.
- Simmer for 10–15 minutes.
- Strain the mixture into a mug and stir in the honey or maple syrup and lemon juice.

Reishi Mushroom Soup:

Ingredients:

- 4 cups bone broth or stock
- ½ cup chopped reishi mushrooms
- 2 cloves of garlic, minced
- 1 tbsp olive oil
- Salt and pepper

Instructions:

- Soak the dried reishi mushrooms in warm water for 20 minutes.
- In a large saucepan, heat the olive oil over medium heat.
- Add the minced garlic and sauté until fragrant.
- Drain the soaked mushrooms and add them to the saucepan with the garlic.
- Add the bone broth or stock and bring to a boil.

- Reduce the heat to low and simmer for 30 minutes, or until the mushrooms are tender.
- Season with salt and pepper to taste.

Maca Energy Balls:

Ingredients:

- 1 cup rolled oats
- ½ cup nut butter (almond butter, peanut butter, etc.)
- ⅓ cup natural sweetener (honey or maple syrup)
- 2 tbsp maca powder
- ¼ cup dark chocolate or unsweetened carob chips

Instructions:

- Combine the rolled oats, nut butter, natural sweetener, and maca powder.
- Mix until well combined.
- Fold in the dark chocolate or unsweetened carob chips.
- Using your hands, roll the mixture into small balls.
- Line a baking pan with parchment paper.
- Place the balls on the baking sheet 1 inch apart and refrigerate for 1 hour.

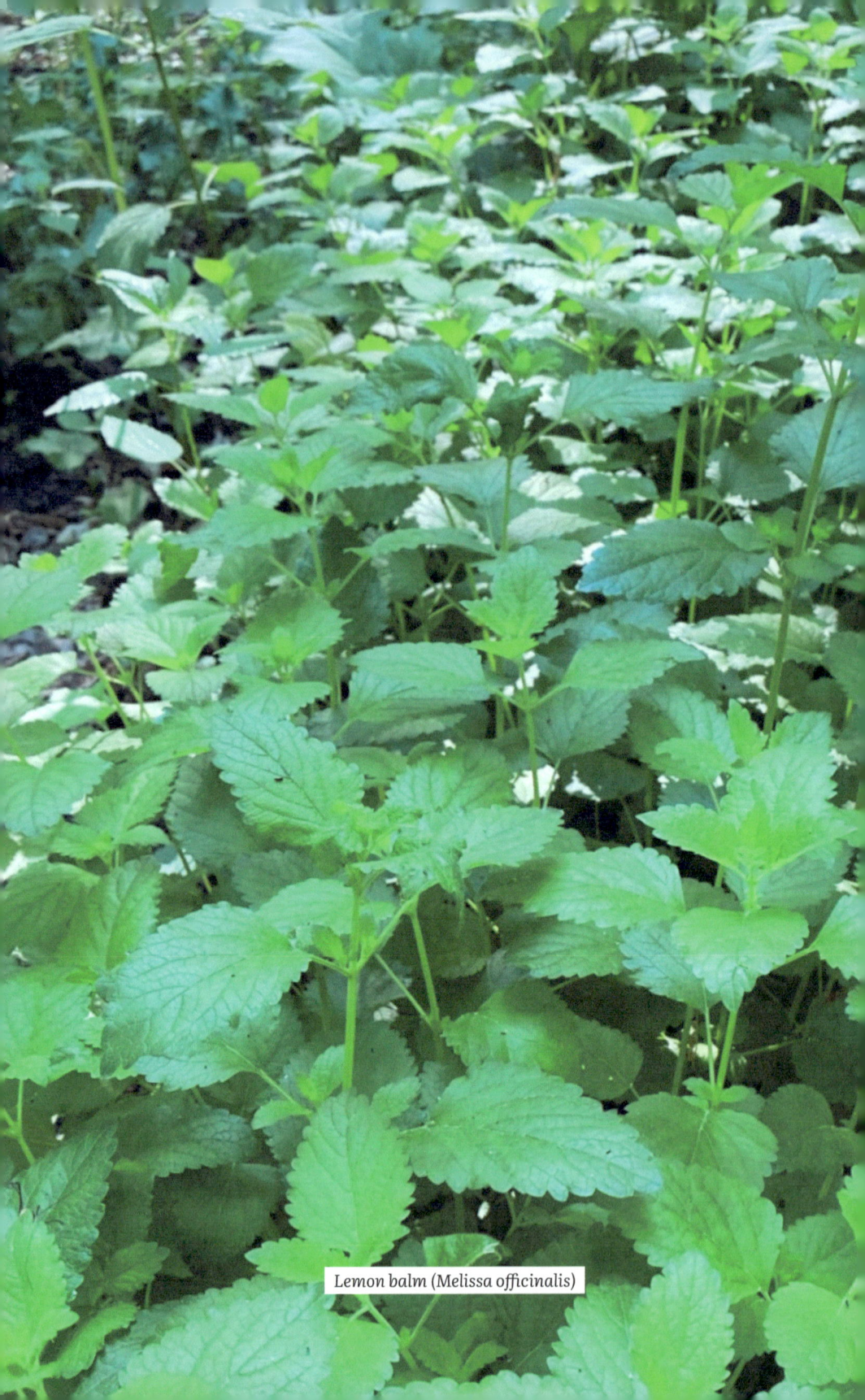
Lemon balm (Melissa officinalis)

CHAPTER 8.
SEDATIVE HERBS

Herbal sedatives are natural remedies that help to promote relaxation, reduce anxiety and stress, and induce sleep without causing harmful side effects. They work by interacting with the body's nervous system and brain chemistry to promote a sense of calm and relaxation. Sedative herbs can be useful for people who suffer from insomnia, anxiety, stress, and other conditions that disrupt sleep or cause nervousness.

Sedative herbs contain compounds that bind to GABA-A receptors in the brain. GABA is a neurotransmitter that produces a calming effect on the nervous system. A good example of one of these compounds is called humulene, found in hops, and when humulene binds to its receptors, it increases the activity of GABA in the brain. This triggers a decrease of activity in the central nervous system and increases activity in the parasympathetic system, resulting in feelings of relaxation and drowsiness.

These herbs can be taken in the form of teas, tinctures, capsules, or tablets.

A) Hops (Humulus lupulus)
B) Skullcap (Scutellaria lateriflora)
C) Chamomile (Matricaria chamomilla
D) Valerian root (Valeriana officinalis)
E) Passionflower (Passiflora incarnata)
F) Lemon balm (Melissa officinalis)

Preparation and dosage

Hops (Humulus lupulus)

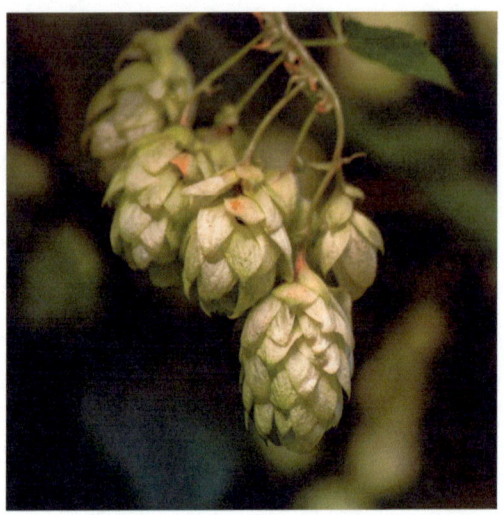

Hops contains two sedative compounds, humulene and methyl-3-buten-2-ol, and when they bind to its receptors, it increases the activity of GABA in the brain promoting a calm and restful sleep.

Hops provides relief for some of the symptoms associated with the flu, as it has been traditionally used as a natural remedy for fever due to its diaphoretic properties. Its anti-inflammatory compounds provide relief by reducing pain and inflammation associated with the flu, such as sore throat, cough, and muscle aches, and its sedative effect may help reduce anxiety and promote restful sleep, which can ease discomfort and help the body fight off an infection faster.

Hops Infusion Recipe:

- Add 2 teaspoons of dried hop cones to a tea ball or tea bag.
- Place in a mug and pour simmering water over the herbs.
- Steep for 5 minutes, then take out the cones.
- Add honey or maple syrup and lemon if desired.
- Drink 1-3 cups of hops tea per day as needed.

Hops Tincture Recipe:

- Place dried hop cones in a jar and cover.

- Pour in enough alcohol to cover, leaving space at the top.*
- Tightly seal the jar, label, date, and shake well.
- Let it steep for 2–3 months. Shake the jar weekly.
- Strain the mixture, then store it in a glass jar in a dark place.
- Take 10–15 drops diluted in a little bit of water up to three times per day as needed.

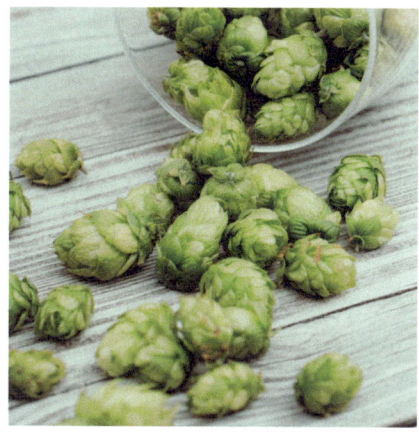

- For children, the proper amount will vary depending on their age and weight. Use 5–7 drops diluted in a small amount of juice or water up to three times a day as needed.

Hops Capsules:

- Hop extract is also available commercially in capsules. Follow the directions for usage on the label.

Note: Excessive use of hops may lead to unwanted side effects, especially in those with hormone-related conditions such as breast cancer, endometriosis, or uterine fibroids. Always consult with a clinical herbalist or health care professional before taking herbal remedies, particularly if you have a health-related condition or are taking medication.

Skullcap (Scutellaria lateriflora)

Skullcap contains flavonoids such as baicalin that have been shown to have sedative effects. These flavonoids bind to certain receptors in the brain, such as GABA-A receptors, involved in the regulation of sleep and anxiety. By binding to these receptors, skullcap helps to increase the levels of the neurotransmitter GABA, which triggers the parasympathetic system and produces a calming effect on the nervous system to promote relaxation and sleep. Skullcap also has mild analgesic properties that can help to alleviate pain and discomfort, further promoting relaxation and restfulness.

Skullcap is primarily known for its calming and relaxing effects, which may indirectly help to reduce pain and discomfort throughout the body that are caused by viruses which trigger stress and tension. In addition, its anti-inflammatory and analgesic properties may help alleviate pain and inflammation in the body.

Skullcap Infusion Recipe:

- Add 2 teaspoons of dried skullcap to a tea ball or tea bag.
- Put in a mug and pour simmering water over the skullcap.
- Steep for 5–10 minutes.
- Remove the herbs.
- Add honey or maple syrup and lemon if desired.
- Drink 1–2 cups of skullcap tea per day as needed.

Skullcap Tincture Recipe:

- Fill a jar with dried skullcap.
- Pour in enough alcohol to cover, leaving space at the top.*
- Tightly seal the jar, label, date, and shake well.
- Let it steep for 2–3 months. Shake the jar weekly.
- Strain the tincture through cheesecloth.
- Pour the tincture back into the jar and store in a dark place.
- Take 10–15 drops diluted in a small amount of water up to three times per day as needed.
- For children, the proper amount will vary depending on their age and weight. Use 5–7 drops diluted in a small amount of juice or water up to three times a day as needed.

Note: Skullcap should not be used by women who are pregnant or breastfeeding. It may also be contraindicated with certain medications such as sedatives and blood thinners. Always consult with a clinical herbalist or health care professional before taking herbal remedies, particularly if you have a health-related condition or are taking medication.

Chamomile (Matricaria chamomilla)

Chamomile contains certain compounds such as apigenin that act on the nervous system to produce a mild sedative effect. Apigenin binds to GABA-A receptors in the brain and triggers the parasympathetic system, causing a calming and relaxing effect on the body that can promote better sleep and relieve anxiety and stress.

Chamomile Infusion Recipe:

- Put 4 teaspoons of fresh chamomile flowers OR 2 teaspoons of dried chamomile flowers into a tea ball or tea bag.
- Place it into a mug and pour simmering water over the flowers.
- Steep for 5–10 minutes.
- Remove the herbs.
- Add honey or maple syrup and lemon if desired.
- Enjoy up to four times a day as needed (or twice a day for children).

Chamomile Tincture Recipe:

- Fill a clean glass jar with dried chamomile flowers.
- Pour in enough alcohol to cover, leaving space at the top.*
- Tightly seal the jar, label, date, and shake well.
- Let it steep for 2–3 months. Shake the jar weekly.
- Strain it through cheesecloth and pour back into the jar.
- Store in a jar in a dark place.
- Take 10–20 drops diluted in a small amount of water up to three times per day as needed.
- For children, the proper amount will vary depending on their age and weight. Use 5–7 drops diluted in a small amount of juice or water up to three times a day as needed.

Note: Always consult with a clinical herbalist or health care professional before taking herbal remedies, particularly if you have a health-related condition or are taking medication.

Valerian Root (Valeriana officinalis)

Valerian root is believed to work as a sedative due to the compounds valerenic acid and valeranone that have been shown to influence the GABA receptors in the brain. When activated, these neurotransmitters help regulate brain activity, promote relaxation, and produce a calming and sedative effect. This can help to reduce anxiety, promote sleep, and relieve tension in the muscles.

Valerian Root Decoction Recipe:

- Bring a pot of water to a boil, then reduce to a simmer.
- Add 1 tablespoon of fresh valerian root OR 1 teaspoon of dried valerian root.
- Cover and let simmer for 10 minutes.
- Take off heat and steep for another 10 minutes.
- Strain the tea and drink.
- Drink 1–3 cups per day as needed.

Valerian Root Tincture Recipe:

- Chop or grind 1 cup of fresh valerian root OR crush ½ cup of dried valerian root and place in a jar.
- Pour in enough alcohol to cover, leaving space at the top.*
- Tightly seal the jar, label, date, and shake well.
- Let it steep for 2–3 months. Shake the jar weekly.
- Strain the liquid through cheesecloth.
- Store the tincture in a clean glass jar and store in a dark place.
- Take 10–15 drops diluted in a little bit of water or juice up to three times a day as needed.
- Valerian root tincture should only be used for children under the advice of a clinical herbalist or health care provider.

Note: Valerian root should not be taken for prolonged periods of time, as it may cause headaches, dizziness, upset stomach, or other side effects. It should also not be taken with alcohol or sedative medications. Pregnant and breastfeeding women should abstain from using valerian root. Always consult with a clinical herbalist or health care professional before taking herbal remedies, particularly if you have a health-related condition or are taking medication.

Passionflower (Passiflora incarnata)

Passionflower is an herbal sedative that works through the GABA neurotransmitters, resulting in a calming effect on the nervous system by triggering the parasympathetic system to help reduce anxiety and promote relaxation. Passionflower contains also compounds called harmala alkaloids that have been shown to have sedative effects, and its flavonoids have antioxidant compounds that may contribute to its sedative effects. These compounds are believed to help reduce inflammation and oxidative stress attributed to the side effects from viruses that cause stress, fatigue, and anxiety. Passionflower has a calming effect on the entire body and promotes relaxation.

Passionflower Infusion Recipe:

- Put 1 tablespoon fresh passionflower OR 1 teaspoon dried passionflower in a tea ball.
- Place in a mug and pour simmering water over the herbs.
- Steep for 5 minutes.
- Strain and enjoy.
- Drink 1–2 cups of passionflower tea per day as needed.

Passionflower Tincture Recipe:

- Fill a jar with dried passionflower.
- Pour in enough alcohol to cover, leaving space at the top.*
- Tightly seal the jar, label, date, and shake well.

- Let it steep for 2–3 months. Shake the jar weekly.
- Strain the tincture through cheesecloth.
- Store the tincture in a glass jar in a dark place.
- Take 10–15 drops diluted in a small amount of water up to three times a day as needed.
- For children, the proper amount will vary depending on their age and weight. Use 5–7 drops diluted in a small amount of juice or water up to three times a day as needed.

Note: As with many herbal remedies, it is recommended to start with a smaller dose and build up with your body's tolerance over time. High doses of passionflower may cause nausea, vomiting, or other adverse effects. Passionflower may cause drowsiness and should not be taken with other sedatives or depressants, including alcohol. It may also be contraindicated with certain medications, including those for anxiety and depression. Always consult with a clinical herbalist or health care professional before taking herbal remedies, particularly if you have a health-related condition or are taking medication.

Lemon Balm (Melissa Officinalis)

Lemon balm is believed to work as a sedative that increases the levels of GABA in the brain, reducing the activity in the autonomic nervous system and promoting relaxation. Lemon balm is also believed to have a mild anti-anxiety effect that further contributes to its sedative properties. It is a very mild sedative that also has a calming effect on fatigue.

Lemon Balm Infusion Recipe:

This tea is refreshing and cooling on hot summer days. Enjoy it as an iced tea throughout the summer.

For iced tea:

- Add 2 handfuls of fresh lemon balm to a pot of simmered water.
- Steep for 10 minutes.
- Strain and refrigerate.

For hot tea:

- Bring 2 cups of water to a boil, then reduce to a simmer.
- Chop ¼ cup of fresh lemon balm leaves (dried leaves loose the aromatic oil) and add the herbs to the water.
- Steep for 5–10 minutes, then strain.
- Add honey or maple syrup and lemon if desired.
- Drink 1–3 mugs of hot lemon balm or 1–3 glasses of iced tea per day as needed.

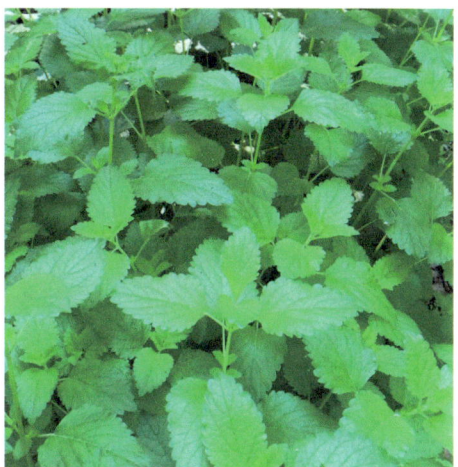

Lemon Balm Tincture Recipe:

- Fill a clean glass jar with fresh lemon balm leaves (dried leaves lose their aromatic oil).
- Pour in enough alcohol to cover, leaving space at the top.*
- Tightly seal the jar, label, date, and shake well.
- Store the jar in a cool place for 2–3 months, shaking the jar weekly.
- Strain the liquid through cheesecloth.
- Pour the tincture into a clean jar and store in a dark place.
- Take 15–20 drops diluted in a little bit of water up to three times per day as needed.
- For children, the proper amount will vary depending on their age and weight. Use 5–7 drops diluted in a small amount of juice or water up to three times a day as needed.

Note: Lemon balm is considered safe when used as directed, but it may cause mild side effects in some people including headache, dizziness, and gastrointestinal upset. It may also be contraindicated with certain medications, including thyroid hormone replacement therapy and sedatives. As with any herbal remedy, it is best to slowly increase the amount used over time and monitor your body's response. Always consult with a clinical herbalist or health care professional before taking herbal remedies, particularly if you have a health-related condition or are taking medication.

Food and Recipes with Calming Effects

- Chamomile is known for its calming properties and can help promote better sleep.
- Warm milk contains the amino acid tryptophan, which can help promote the production of melatonin, a sleep hormone.
- Bananas contain magnesium, which can help relax muscles and promote a sense of calm.
- Oatmeal is a complex carbohydrate that can increase the production of serotonin, which promotes a calming effect.
- Almonds are rich in magnesium, which can help relax muscles and promote a sense of calm.

Chamomile and Banana Smoothie:

- Blend together 1 frozen banana, 1 cup of non-dairy or cow's milk, ¼ cup of rolled oats, 1 tsp of honey, and chilled chamomile tea.
- Serve cold.

Warm Milk:

- Heat 1 cup of cow's milk or non-dairy unsweetened almond or coconut milk on the stove until warm.
- Stir in 1 tsp of maple syrup or honey and ¼ tsp of cinnamon.
- Enjoy before bedtime.

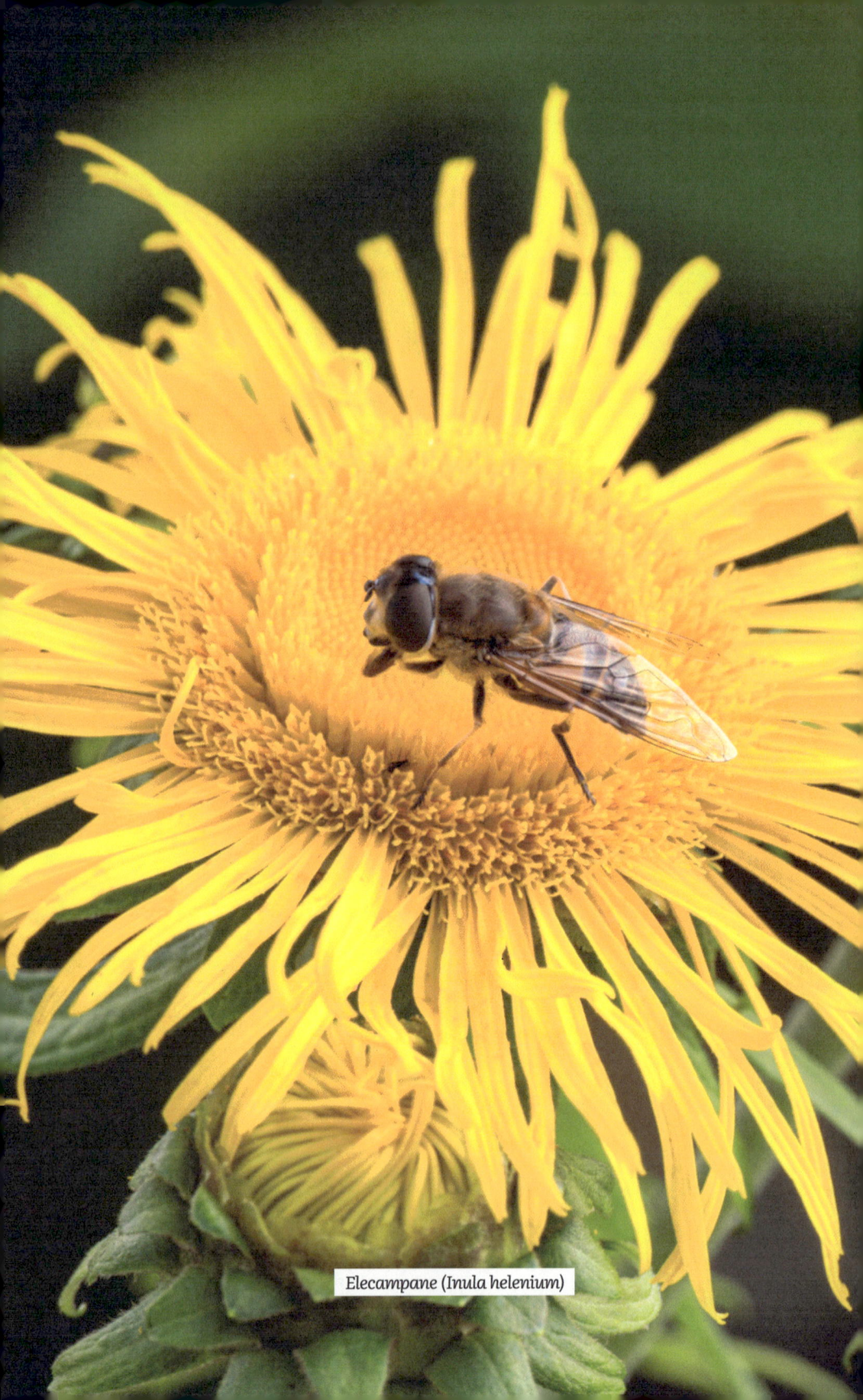
Elecampane (Inula helenium)

CHAPTER 9.
BITTER STOMACHIC HERBS

Stomachic herbs promote good digestion by stimulating the production of digestive enzymes and promoting proper bile flow, thus relieving symptoms of indigestion, bloating, and gas.

Some stomachic herbs have an anti-inflammatory effect that may reduce inflammation in the digestive tract, leading to improved gut health, while others have a calming effect that may help alleviate symptoms of stress and anxiety that can contribute to digestive issues.

Certain stomachic herbs help relieve spasms in the digestive tract and may reduce the symptoms of irritable bowel syndrome (IBS). Others have anti-microbial properties that can help eliminate destructive bacteria in the gut and support improved gut health.

A) Chamomile (Matricaria chamomilla)
B) Ginger (Zingiber officinale)
C) Peppermint (Mentha piperita)
D) Codonopsis (Codonopsis pilosula)
E) Elecampane (Inula helenium)
F) Gentian (Gentiana lutea)
G) Turmeric (Curcuma longa)
H) Licorice (Glycyrrhiza glabra)
I) Yellow dock root (Rumex crispus)

Preparation & Dosage

Chamomile (Matricaria chamomilla)

Chamomile is a popular herb that has been used for centuries as a digestive aid. It works as a stomachic herb through its anti-inflammatory, antispasmodic, and carminative properties.

- Chamomile contains compounds that have anti-inflammatory effects on the digestive system, helping to reduce inflammation and irritation in the stomach and intestines.
- Chamomile has antispasmodic effects, meaning it can help to relax the muscles in the digestive system and reduce cramping and spasms.
- Chamomile also has carminative properties that may help reduce gas and bloating in the digestive system. This is especially beneficial for people who experience flatulence and abdominal discomfort after meals.

Chamomile Infusion Recipe:

- Place 3 teaspoons of chamomile flowers into a tea ball or tea bag into a mug.
- Place in a mug and pour simmering water over the flowers.
- Steep for 5–10 minutes.
- Add honey or maple syrup and lemon if desired.
- Drink 1–3 cups of chamomile tea per day after meals as needed.

Chamomile Tincture Recipe:

- Fill a jar with dried chamomile flowers.
- Pour in enough alcohol to cover, leaving space at the top.*
- Tightly seal the jar, label, date, and shake well.
- Let it steep for 2–3 months. Shake the jar weekly.
- Strain the mixture through cheesecloth.

- Store in a jar in a dark place.
- Take 8–10 drops diluted in a small amount of water up to three times a day as needed.
- For children, the proper amount will vary depending on their age and weight. Use 5–7 drops diluted in a small amount of juice or water up to three times a day as needed to promote digestion and encourage a good night's sleep.

Note: Always consult with a clinical herbalist or health care professional before taking herbal remedies, particularly if you have a health-related condition or are taking medication.

Ginger (Zingiber officinale)

Ginger has been used in many cultures throughout history as a digestive aid. Ginger works as a stomachic herb and has anti-inflammatory, carminative, and digestive stimulant properties.

- Ginger's anti-inflammatory compounds have positive effects on the digestive system, helping to reduce inflammation and irritation in the stomach and intestines.
- Ginger may help to reduce gas and bloating in the digestive system. Ginger's carminative actions may reduce flatulence and abdominal discomfort after meals.
- Ginger also acts as a digestive stimulant, helping to increase the production of digestive enzymes.

Ginger Infusion Recipe:

- Bring 2 cups of water to a boil.
- Cut fresh ginger root into thin slices OR use 2 teaspoons of dried ginger root.
- Add ginger to the boiling water and cover the pot.
- Reduce heat and let simmer for 10 minutes.
- Remove from heat, then strain.

- Add honey or maple syrup and lemon if desired.
- Drink 1–2 mugs of ginger per day after a meal as needed.

For nausea or vomiting, ginger tea can be consumed as needed up to three times per day.

Ginger Tincture Recipe:

- Fill a jar with chopped fresh ginger root or dried ginger.
- Pour in enough alcohol to cover, leaving space at the top.*
- Tightly seal the jar, label, date, and shake well.
- Let it steep for 2–3 months. Shake the jar weekly.
- Strain the mixture through cheesecloth.
- Store the tincture in a jar in a dark place.
- Take 10 drops diluted in a small amount of water up to three times per day as needed. For nausea or vomiting, ginger tincture can be taken as needed, up to three times per day.
- For children, the proper amount will vary depending on their age and weight. Use 3–5 drops diluted in a small amount of juice or water up to three times a day as needed.

Note: Always consult with a clinical herbalist or health care professional before taking herbal remedies, particularly if you have a health-related condition or are taking medication.

Peppermint (Mentha piperita)

Peppermint as a digestive aid has a long history of use. Peppermint's action as a stomachic herb has the potential to relax smooth muscles in the digestive tract, stimulate the secretion of digestive juices, and reduce inflammation in the gut. Peppermint contains menthol, an aromatic essential oil proven to have antispasmodic and analgesic effects. This makes peppermint a useful herb for the digestive system to relieve symptoms of indigestion, bloating, and stomach cramps.

Peppermint Infusion Recipe:

- Place 2 tablespoons of chopped fresh peppermint leaves OR 2 teaspoons of dried peppermint leaves into a tea ball or infuser.
- Place in a mug and pour simmering water over the peppermint.
- Let the peppermint steep for 5–10 minutes.
- Strain the leaves.
- Add honey or maple syrup and lemon if desired.
- Drink 2–3 mugs per day after meals or as needed.

Peppermint Tincture Recipe:

- Fill a clean glass jar with dried or fresh peppermint leaves.
- Pour in enough alcohol to cover, leaving space at the top.*
- Tightly seal the jar, label, date, and shake well.
- Let it steep for 2–3 months. Shake the jar weekly.
- Strain the tincture through cheesecloth.
- Store the tincture in a clean glass jar in a dark place.
- Take 10–15 drops diluted in a little bit of water up to three times per day as needed.
- For children, the proper amount will vary depending on their age and weight. Use 5–7 drops diluted in a small amount of juice or water up to two times a day as needed.

Note: Avoid using peppermint essential oil internally, as it can be toxic. Peppermint may be contraindicated with certain medications and may cause side effects in some individuals. Always consult with a clinical herbalist or health care professional before taking herbal remedies, particularly if you have a health-related condition or are taking medication.

Codonopsis (Codonopsis pilosula)

Codonopsis, also known as dang shen, is considered an effective stomach tonic in TCM. It is believed to help regulate digestive functions and improve nutrient absorption as well as stimulate the production of digestive enzymes. In TCM, Codonopsis is believed to tone the spleen and lungs, promote digestion, and increase energy and vitality. It is also believed to have immune-boosting properties and is often used to support respiratory health.

Codonopsis Decoction Recipe:

- Bring 2 cups of water to a boil, then reduce to a simmer.
- Chop 2 teaspoons dried codonopsis root and add to the simmering water.
- Cover and simmer for 10 minutes.
- Turn off the heat and steep for another 5 minutes.
- Strain the mixture.
- Add natural sweetener and lemon if desired.
- Drink up to three cups per day as needed after meals.

Codonopsis Tincture Recipe:

- Fill a jar with dried codonopsis root.
- Pour in enough alcohol to cover, leaving space at the top.*
- Tightly seal the jar, label, date, and shake well.
- Let it steep for 2–3 months. Shake the jar weekly.
- Strain the mixture through cheesecloth.
- Store the tincture in a clean glass jar in a cool place.
- Take 10–15 drops diluted in a small amount of water up to three times per day as needed.

Note: Codonopsis is considered safe as a food and as an herbal remedy in recommended doses. However, it may cause side effects in some people, such as upset stomach, diarrhea, and allergic reactions. Always consult with a clinical herbalist or health care professional before taking herbal remedies, particularly if you have a health-related condition or are taking medication.

Elecampane (Inula helenium)

Elecampane is a good stomach herb due to its high concentration of bitter compounds known as sesquiterpene lactones. These bitter compounds stimulate the production and secretion of digestive enzymes, which help to improve digestion, relieve the symptoms bloating, gas, and constipation. Elecampane is also rich in inulin, a prebiotic fiber that helps support the growth of beneficial gut bacteria, further improving digestive health.

Besides Elecampanes benefits for digestive issues it has antimicrobial properties, which support the immune system for respiratory infections such as bronchitis, pneumonia, coughs, and other conditions related to the lungs and respiratory system.

Elecampane Decoction Recipe:

- Bring 4 cups of water to a boil, then reduce to a simmer.
- Add 2 tablespoons of chopped fresh elecampane root OR dried elecampane root to the simmering water.
- Cover and simmer for 5–10 minutes.
- Strain the mixture.
- Add honey and lemon if desired.
- Drink slowly (2 ounces at a time up) and enjoy up to two cups per day as needed.

Start with drinking 2 ounces and gradually increase the amount as needed while paying attention to how your body responds.

Elecampane Tincture Recipe:

- Fill a glass jar with chopped elecampane root.
- Pour in enough alcohol to cover, leaving space at the top.*
- Tightly seal the jar, label, date, and shake well.
- Let it steep for 2–3 months. Shake the jar weekly.
- Strain the mixture through cheesecloth.

- Pour the tincture into a glass jar and store in a dark place.
- Take 20–30 drops diluted in a small amount of water or juice up to three times per day as needed.
- For children, the proper amount will vary depending on their age and weight. Use 5–7 drops diluted in a small amount of juice or water up to three times a day as needed.

Note: Elecampane may be contraindicated with certain medications and is not recommended for use during pregnancy or breastfeeding. Always consult with a clinical herbalist or health care professional before taking herbal remedies, particularly if you have a health-related condition or are taking medication.

Gentian (Gentiana lutea)

Gentian root contains bitter compounds such as gentiopicrin that are known to stimulate the production of digestive juices and enzymes in the stomach, liver, and pancreas. This activity helps improve digestion, stimulate appetite, and relieve bloating, gas, and nausea. Gentian has anti-inflammatory and antibacterial properties as well that may help the digestive tract and prevent infections.

Gentian Infusion Recipe:

- Bring 2 cups of water to a boil.
- Add 1 teaspoon of dried gentian root and cover the pot.
- Reduce heat and simmer for 5–10 minutes.
- Strain the tea.
- Add honey and lemon if desired.
- Drink hot. Drink 2 ounces at a time and enjoy up to two cups per day as needed.

Gentian Tincture Recipe:

- Chop the gentian root into small pieces and place in a jar.
- Pour in enough alcohol to cover, leaving space at the top.*
- Tightly seal the jar, label, date, and shake well.
- Let it steep for 2–3 months. Shake the jar weekly.
- Strain the mixture through cheesecloth.
- Store the tincture in a glass jar in a dark place.
- Take 10–15 drops diluted with a little bit of water up to three times per day as needed.
- For children, the proper amount will vary depending on their age and weight. Use 5–7 drops diluted in a small amount of juice or water up to three times a day as needed.

Note: Gentian may be contraindicated with certain medications, such as blood thinners or antihypertensive drugs. It should not be used if you are pregnant, breastfeeding, or have gastric or duodenal ulcers. Always consult with a clinical herbalist or health care professional before taking herbal remedies, particularly if you have a health-related condition or are taking medication.

Turmeric (Curcuma longa)

Turmeric's powerful curcumin compound is an anti-inflammatory that helps reduce inflammation in the stomach and digestive system.

Turmeric Decoction Recipe:

- Bring 2 cups of water to a boil.
- Add 1 teaspoon of chopped or powdered turmeric, turn down the heat, and cover the pot.
- Simmer for 5–10 minutes.
- Add honey and lemon to taste if desired.
- Drink up to three cups per day as needed.

Turmeric Tincture Recipe:

- Wash 1 cup of fresh turmeric root and chop it into small pieces. Place in a jar.
- Pour in enough alcohol to cover, leaving space at the top.*
- Tightly seal the jar, label, date, and shake well.
- Let it steep for 2–3 months. Shake the jar weekly.
- Strain the mixture, then store it in a glass jar in a dark place.
- Take 15–20 drops diluted in a little bit of water up to three times per day as needed.
- For children, the proper amount will vary depending on their age and weight. Use 5–7 drops diluted in a small amount of juice or water up to three times a day as needed.

Note: Always consult with a clinical herbalist or health care professional before taking herbal remedies, particularly if you have a health-related condition or are taking medication.

Licorice (Glycyrrhiza glabra)

Licorice has many actions that support the immune system. When a virus settles in with symptoms of the common cold or the flu, it begins to weaken our health. Acute symptoms of the flu tend to be more severe and can lead to serious complications such as pneumonia. However, self-care using licorice blended with other herbal remedies may very well wipe out the cold, flu, and pneumonia.

- As a demulcent, the protective coating soothes inflammation in the mucus membranes of the stomach, intestines, and the throat.
- As an expectorant, licorice loosens and expels mucus from the respiratory system and the intestines.
- As an antiviral, licorice treats infections, and its anti-inflammatory compounds provide some comfort by reducing inflammation throughout the body.

- As a digestive aid, licorice stimulates digestive function and may reduce inflammation by soothing stomach aches and acid reflux. Licorice also contains glycyrrhizin, an anti-inflammatory and antioxidant that may help reduce inflammation in the stomach and intestines.

Licorice Root Decoction Recipe:

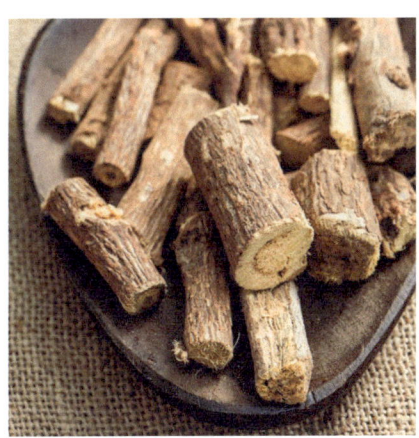

- Bring 2 cups of water to a boil.
- Add 1 tablespoon of dried licorice root, cover, and turn the heat down to a simmer.
- Reduce the heat to low and let the mixture simmer for 10–15 minutes.
- Strain the tea.
- Add lemon if desired.
- Enjoy up to twice a day as needed either hot or chilled (or once a day for children).

Licorice Root Tincture Recipe:

- Crush 1 cup of dried licorice root using a mortar and pestle or a food processor. Place the crushed licorice root in a glass jar.
- Pour in enough alcohol to cover, leaving space at the top.*
- Tightly seal the jar, label, date, and shake well.
- Let it steep for 2–3 months. Shake the jar weekly.
- Strain through cheesecloth or a coffee filter.
- Pour the tincture into a glass jar and store it in a cool place.
- Take 7–10 drops diluted in a little bit of water up to three times per day as needed.
- For children, the proper amount will vary depending on their age and weight. Use 5–7 drops diluted in a small amount of juice or water up to two times a day as needed.

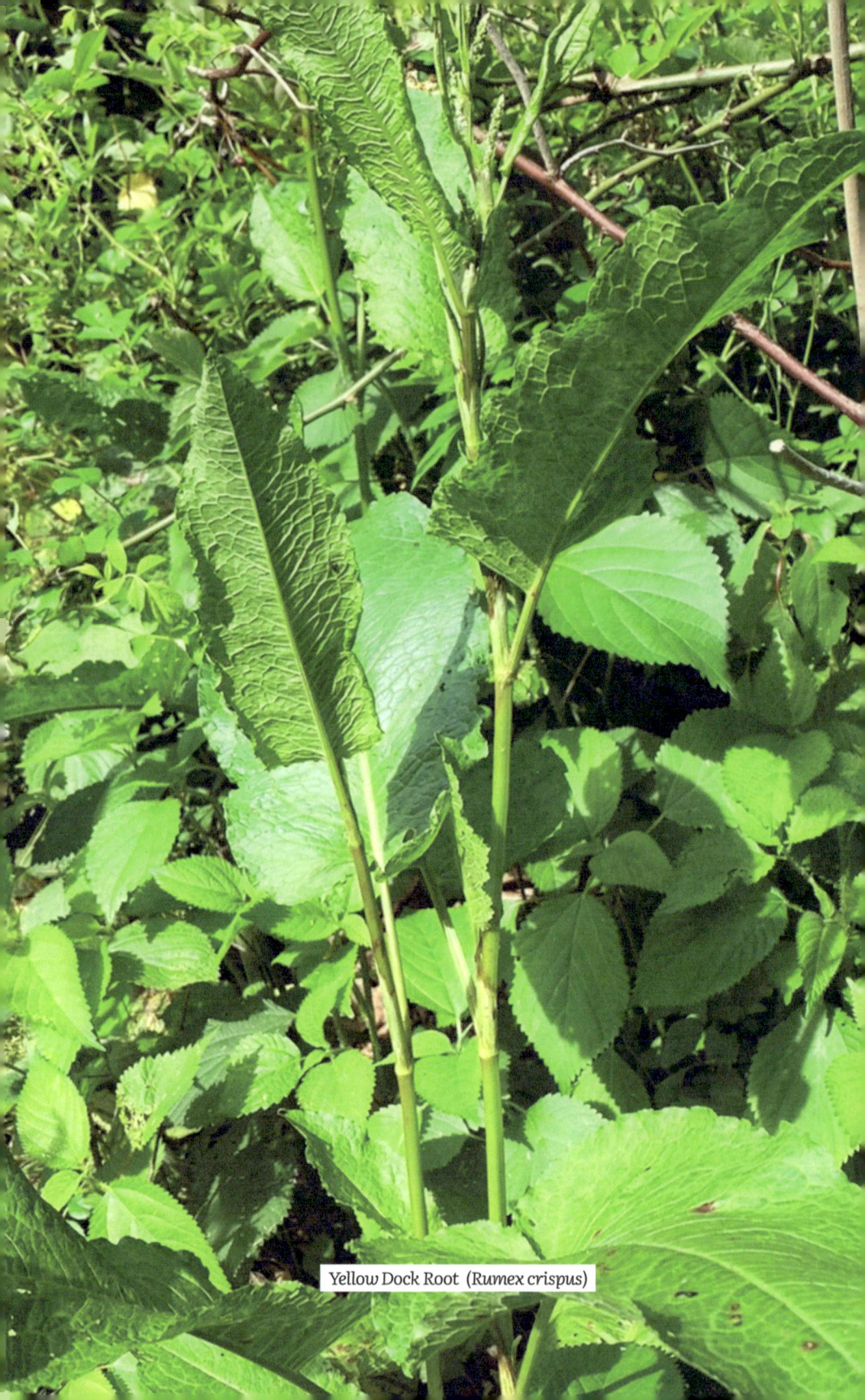
Yellow Dock Root (*Rumex crispus*)

Note: Always consult with a clinical herbalist or health care professional before taking herbal remedies, particularly if you have a health-related condition or are taking medication.

Yellow Dock Root (Rumex crispus)

Yellow dock root is a bitter herb that stimulates the production of digestive enzymes needed for healthy digestion. The beneficial action comes from the compound anthraquinone that increases bile flow. It is also known to have anti-inflammatory compounds that help reduce inflammation of the digestive tract.

Yellow dock root is a good source of potassium as well as other minerals, vitamins, and antioxidants that support and regulate the fluids in the body. The antioxidant actions have detoxifying benefits that encourage the proper functions of a healthy colon and liver.

Regular consumption of yellow dock root will boost the production of bile and stimulate the detoxification process of the liver and colon necessary for a healthy digestive system. It supports the flow of bile from the liver to the gallbladder to the colon, which is needed to digest, metabolize, and eliminate food. It also tones the colon and normalizes bowel functions, eliminating constipation and diarrhea.

Lastly, since yellow dock contains iron, it is an excellent herb for mild anemia caused by iron deficiency. It collects iron from the earth and combines it with the minerals and vitamins needed for the body to effectively absorb iron.

Yellow Dock Root Decoction Recipe:

- Boil 2 cups of water.
- Add 2 teaspoons of chopped yellow dock root, turn down the heat, and cover.
- Simmer for 10–15 minutes.

- Strain the mixture.
- Drink two ounces at a time and enjoy up to two mugs per day as needed.
- As a supplement for normal bowel functions, drink 2 ounces per day.

Yellow Dock Root Tincture Recipe:

- Chop fresh or dried yellow dock root and place in a jar.
- Pour in enough alcohol to cover, leaving space at the top.*
- Tightly seal the jar, label, date, and shake well.
- Let it steep for 2–3 months. Shake the jar weekly.
- Strain the mixture, then store it in a glass jar in a dark place.
- Take 15–20 drops diluted in a small amount of water up to three times a day as needed.
- For children, the proper amount will vary depending on their age and weight. Use 5–7 drops diluted in a small amount of juice or water up to three times a day as needed.

Note: Yellow dock root should not be taken by people that have kidney disease or if you are nursing or breastfeeding. It may also be contraindicated with certain medications. Always consult with a clinical herbalist or health care professional before taking herbal remedies, particularly if you have a health-related condition or are taking medication.

Food and Recipes That Aid Digestion

Ginger Tea:

- Steep fresh ginger slices in a mug of simmering water for a few minutes.

Ginger is known to have anti-inflammatory and anti-spasmodic properties that can help soothe the digestive tract and relieve nausea.

Miso Soup with Tofu and Seaweed:

Miso paste contains probiotics that can help promote a healthy gut microbiome and aid in digestion.

Ingredients:

- 4 cups dashi stock (or vegetable broth for a vegetarian/vegan version)
- 3 tablespoons miso paste (white or red, according to preference)
- ½ cup cubed tofu
- 2 tablespoons dried seaweed (such as wakame), rehydrated in water and drained
- 2 green onions, thinly sliced
- Optional: 1 teaspoon soy sauce or tamari (for added depth of flavor)
- Optional: Sliced mushrooms or other vegetables of your choice

Instructions:

1. Prepare the dashi stock: If using dashi stock granules or powder, follow the package instructions to make 4 cups of dashi stock. If using vegetable broth, heat the broth in a pot over medium heat until simmering.
2. Add the tofu and seaweed: Once the stock is simmering, add the cubed tofu and rehydrated seaweed to the pot. If using mushrooms or other vegetables, add them at this stage as well. Let them simmer for a few minutes until the tofu is heated through and the vegetables are tender.
3. Dilute the miso paste: In a small bowl, dilute the miso paste with a few tablespoons of hot broth from the pot. Stir well until the miso paste is fully dissolved and no clumps remain.
4. Add the miso paste to the soup: Reduce the heat to low and gently stir in the diluted miso paste into the soup. Be careful not to let the soup come to a boil after adding the miso, as high heat

can diminish its flavor. If desired, add soy sauce or tamari for an extra depth of flavor.
5. Serve and garnish: Ladle the miso soup into bowls. Garnish with sliced green onions.
6. Enjoy: Serve the miso soup hot and enjoy its comforting flavors and nourishing qualities. It can be enjoyed as a starter, a side dish, or a light meal on its own.

Note: Miso paste can vary in saltiness, so adjust the amount used according to your taste preference. It is best to taste the soup as you cook and add more miso if desired. Additionally, feel free to customize the soup by adding other ingredients, vegetables, or cooked noodles.

Papaya Salad with Chili Peppers and Lime Juice:

An enzyme in papaya called papain may relieve the symptoms of gout by breaking down proteins in the digestive tract, making it easier to digest food. Chili peppers may also help stimulate digestive juices.

Ingredients:

- 1 green papaya
- 1-2 Thai chili peppers (adjust to your preferred level of spiciness)
- 2 cloves of garlic
- 2 tablespoons fish sauce
- 2 tablespoons fresh lime juice (adjust to taste)
- 1 tablespoon palm sugar or brown sugar
- 1 small tomato, sliced
- 1 handful of green beans, trimmed and cut into bite-sized pieces
- 2 tablespoons crushed peanuts
- Fresh cilantro leaves for garnish
- Optional: shrimp or grilled chicken (for added protein)

Instructions:

1. Peel and shred the green papaya: Cut off the top and bottom of the papaya. Use a peeler to remove the skin. Cut the papaya in half lengthwise and scoop out the seeds. Shred the papaya using a grater or a julienne peeler. Place the shredded papaya in a large mixing bowl.
2. Prepare the dressing: In a mortar and pestle, pound the garlic and Thai chili peppers together until they form a coarse paste. Alternatively, you can mince the garlic and chili peppers finely. Add the fish sauce, lime juice, and palm sugar to the mortar and pestle (or a small bowl) and stir until the sugar dissolves.
3. Toss the salad: Add the dressing to the shredded papaya in the mixing bowl. Use clean hands or tongs to gently mix and massage the papaya with the dressing, ensuring the papaya is evenly coated.
4. Add the remaining ingredients: Add the sliced tomato and green beans to the papaya mixture. Toss to combine.
5. Serve and garnish: Transfer the papaya salad to a serving plate. Sprinkle crushed peanuts over the top. Garnish with fresh cilantro leaves. If desired, you can also add cooked shrimp or grilled chicken for added protein.
6. Enjoy: Serve the papaya salad immediately and enjoy the vibrant flavors and textures of this refreshing dish.

Note: Feel free to adjust the ingredients and seasonings according to your taste preferences. You can add more lime juice for extra tanginess or increase the amount of chili peppers for additional heat.

Yogurt:

Yogurt contains probiotics that can help improve digestion and promote a healthy gut microbiome. Look for brands that specifically advertise the presence of live and active cultures.

Whole Grain Toast with Avocado:

- Smash the flesh of an avocado onto a piece of whole grain toast.

Avocado can aid in digestion because it is high in fiber, which can help promote regular bowel movements. Whole grain toast provides additional fiber and nutrients.

Bone Broth Vegetable Barley Soup:

Bone broth contains nutrients that can help repair gut lining and promote healthy digestion.

Ingredients:

- 1 tablespoon olive oil
- 1 onion, diced
- 2 carrots, diced
- 2 celery stalks, diced
- 2 cloves garlic, minced
- 1 cup diced tomatoes (fresh or canned)
- 1 cup diced potatoes
- ½ cup pearl barley
- 6 cups bone broth (chicken, beef, or vegetable)
- 1 teaspoon dried thyme
- 1 bay leaf
- Salt and pepper to taste
- Chopped fresh parsley for garnish

Instructions:

1. Heat the olive oil in a large pot over medium heat. Add the diced onion, carrots, and celery. Sauté for about 5 minutes until the vegetables start to soften.
2. Add the minced garlic and cook for an additional minute until fragrant.

3. Add the diced tomatoes, potatoes, pearl barley, bone broth, dried thyme, and bay leaf to the pot. Bring the mixture to a boil.
4. Once boiling, reduce the heat to low, cover the pot, and let the soup simmer for about 45 minutes to 1 hour, or until the barley and vegetables are tender.
5. Season the soup with salt and pepper to taste. Adjust the seasonings as needed.
6. Remove the bay leaf from the pot before serving.
7. Ladle the soup into bowls and garnish with chopped fresh parsley.
8. Serve hot and enjoy the nourishing flavors of the bone broth vegetable barley soup.

Note: You can customize this soup by adding other vegetables of your choice, such as peas, corn, or green beans. Feel free to experiment with different herbs and spices to suit your taste preferences. Additionally, bone broth can be homemade or store-bought, depending on your preference and availability.

Roasted Vegetables:

Roasted vegetables are high in fiber and promote regular bowel movements. Roasting them can also help make them easier to digest.

Ingredients:

- Assorted vegetables of your choice (such as carrots, potatoes, sweet potatoes, bell peppers, broccoli, cauliflower, zucchini, etc.)
- Olive oil
- Salt and pepper to taste
- Optional: Herbs or spices of your choice (such as garlic powder, paprika, thyme, rosemary, etc.)

Instructions:

1. Preheat your oven to 425°F (220°C).
2. Wash and prepare the vegetables: Peel and chop the vegetables into similar-sized pieces. Keep in mind that denser vegetables like carrots and potatoes may take longer to cook, so you can cut them into slightly smaller pieces compared to softer vegetables like zucchini or bell peppers.
3. Toss the vegetables with olive oil: In a large bowl, drizzle the vegetables with olive oil. Use enough oil to coat the vegetables evenly but not excessively. Add salt, pepper, and any desired herbs or spices. Toss the vegetables gently to ensure they are well coated.
4. Spread the vegetables onto a baking sheet: Arrange the seasoned vegetables in a single layer on a baking sheet lined with parchment paper or lightly greased. Avoid overcrowding the vegetables, as this can prevent them from roasting evenly.
5. Roast in the oven: Place the baking sheet in the preheated oven and roast the vegetables for about 25–35 minutes, or until they are golden brown and tender. The exact cooking time may vary depending on the size and type of vegetables, so keep an eye on them and stir halfway through the cooking process for even browning.
6. Serve and enjoy: Once the vegetables are roasted to your desired level of doneness, remove them from the oven and transfer them to a serving dish. They are delicious as a side dish or can be used as a base for other recipes. Enjoy the flavorful and caramelized roasted vegetables!

Feel free to customize this recipe by adding your favorite vegetables or experimenting with different herbs and spices. Roasted vegetables are versatile and can be enjoyed as a simple side dish or incorporated into various dishes like salads, grain bowls, pasta, or as toppings for pizzas.

Kefir Smoothie:

- Blend kefir with fruits and vegetables of your choice.

Kefir is a fermented beverage that contains probiotics and promotes a healthy gut microbiome. Blending it into a smoothie with fruits and vegetables provides additional nutrients and fiber.

Everybody's digestive system is different, and what may work for one person may not work for another. Try a little bit of each food group and pay attention to how your body reacts to different foods, then steadily increase your serving size.

CHAPTER 10.
TONIC HERBS

Tonic herbs are plants that are traditionally used to promote overall health and vitality and are believed to have a strengthening and balancing effect on the body. These herbs work by supporting and nourishing the body's natural processes rather than targeting a specific symptom or condition.

Tonic herbs are often rich in nutrients and other bioactive compounds such as antioxidants and adaptogens that may help reduce inflammation, support the immune system, balance hormones, and promote healthy digestion. Some tonic herbs may also have specific benefits for certain organs or systems in the body.

Unlike many conventional medications that may have side effects or risks associated with long-term use, tonic herbs are considered safe for most people and can be used regularly as part of a healthy lifestyle. The effects of tonic herbs may be subtle and cumulative, as it may take time to balance the homeostasis.

A) Nettle (Urtica dioica)
B) Dandelion (Taraxacum officinale)
C) Licorice (Glycyrrhiza glabra)
D) Elecampane (Inula helenium)
E) Coltsfoot (Tussilago farfara)
F) White tea & green tea (Camellia sinensis)

Preparation & Dosage

Nettle (Urtica dioica)

Nettle is a diverse tonic herb with a variety of health benefits. Besides being rich in vitamins and minerals, iron, calcium, magnesium, and vitamins A and C, nettle is considered a safe and beneficial tonic herb that can be used as a daily supplement to support overall health and well-being.

Nettle contains compounds that have immune-boosting properties to help protect against infections as well as anti-inflammatory compounds that help reduce inflammation throughout the body and alleviate conditions such as arthritis and allergies. It has long been used as an herbal remedy in traditional medicine for respiratory conditions such as asthma, bronchitis, and allergies.

As a diuretic, nettle increases urine production and thus helps to flush out toxins from the body. It is also used to support the health of the kidneys and bladder. Nettle has been shown to have positive effects on blood pressure, cholesterol levels, and circulation, giving it the potential to reduce the risk of heart disease.

Nettle Infusion Recipe:

- For dried nettles, add 1 cup of dried nettle leaves to a quart-sized jar.
- Pour simmering water over the nettle. Fill the jar to the top.
- Seal the jar and let it steep overnight or for at least 4 hours.
- Strain and drink 1–2 cups daily as needed.
- For fresh nettles, add 2 cups to a quart of simmering water and simmer with the lid on for 5–10 minutes.
- Strain and drink 1–2 cups daily as needed.

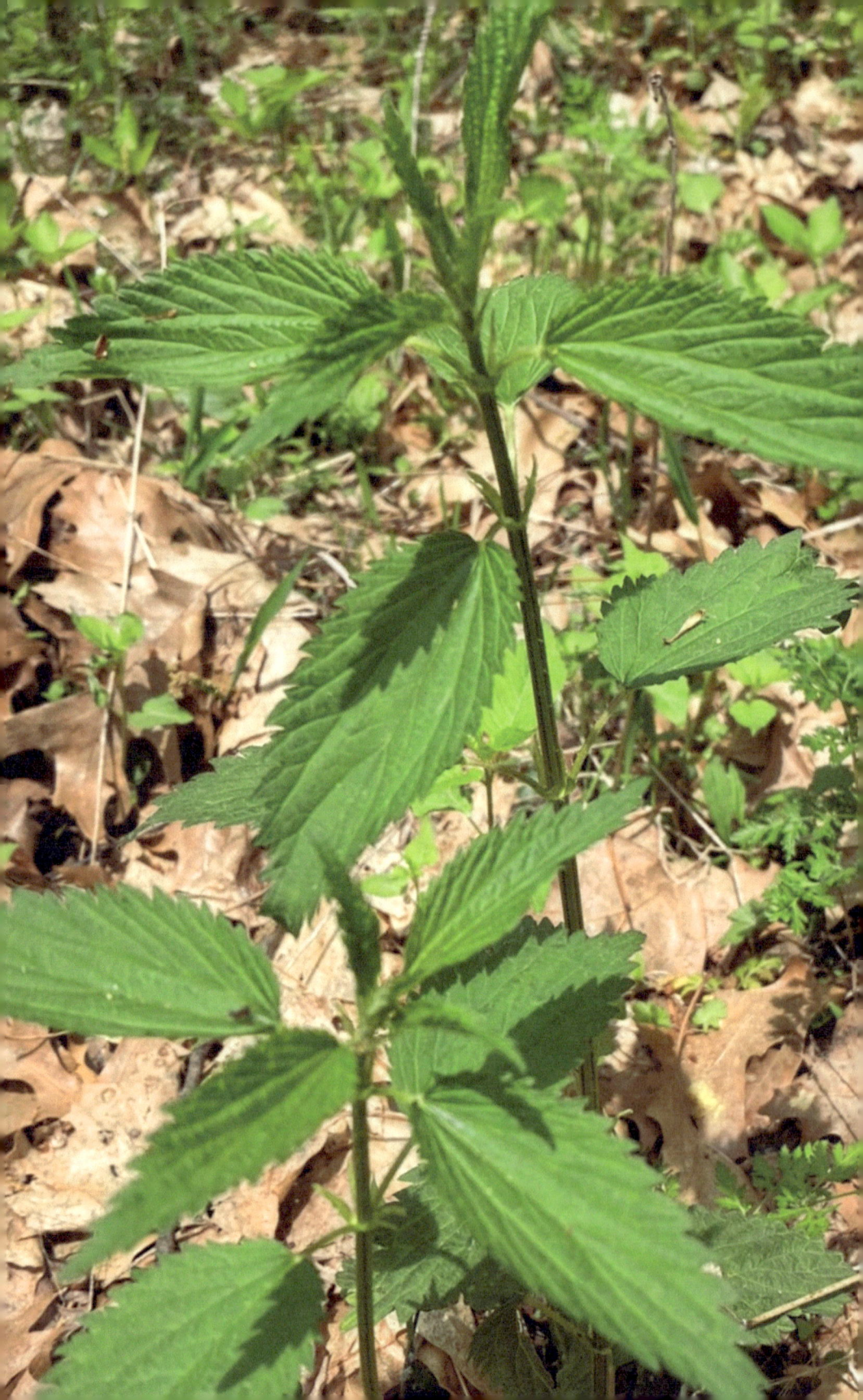

Nettle Tincture Recipe:

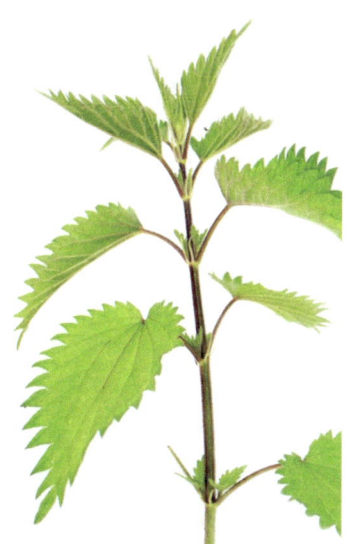

- Fill a jar ⅔ full of dried nettle leaves.
- Pour in enough alcohol to cover, leaving space at the top.*
- Tightly seal the jar, label, date, and shake well.
- Let it steep for 2–3 months. Shake the jar weekly.
- Strain the mixture, then store it in a glass jar in a dark place.
- Take 15–20 drops diluted in a little bit of water up to two times a day as needed.
- For children, the proper amount will vary depending on their age and weight. Use 5–7 drops diluted in a small amount of juice or water once a day as needed.

Nettle Vinegar Recipe:

- Fill a quart-sized jar with fresh nettle leaves.
- Pour raw apple cider vinegar over the leaves until they are completely covered.
- Seal the jar with a non-metallic lid and let it sit in a cool, dark place for 3–6 months.
- Strain the mixture, then store it in a glass bottle in the refrigerator.
- Take 1 tablespoon of vinegar diluted in a small amount of water before meals to support good digestion and as a daily tonic.

Nettles are considered safe for most people; however, some people may be allergic. Drink a couple of ounces of tea to start with and steadily increase the amount if you experience no side effects. Contact with the plant itself can also cause skin irritation; proceed with caution if cutting fresh leaves, as they have stinging nettle hairs on the edges of the leaves.

Note: Nettles may have contraindications with certain medications, including blood thinners, blood pressure medications, and some diabetes medications. It is also important to avoid using nettles if you have a history of kidney stones or kidney disease. Always consult with a clinical herbalist or health care professional before taking herbal remedies, particularly if you have a health-related condition or are taking medication.

Dandelion (Taraxacum officinale)

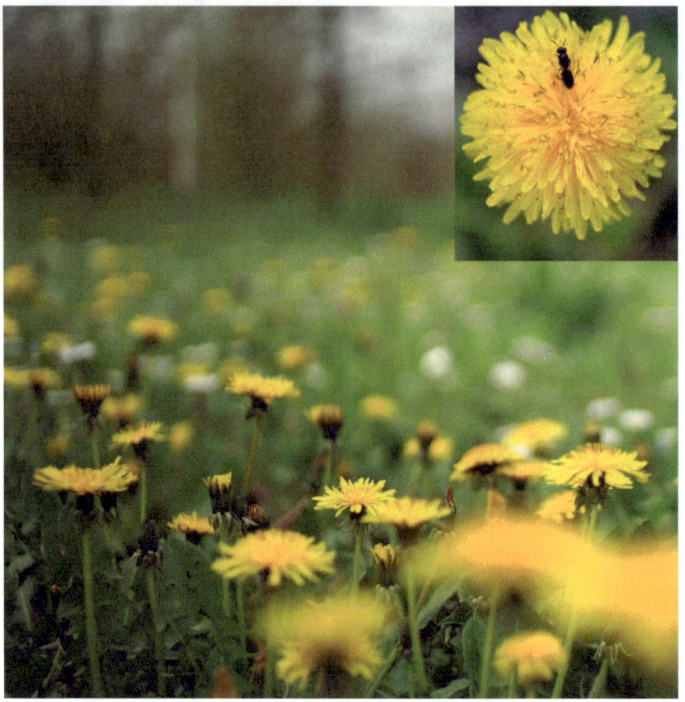

Dandelion's tonic actions work by stimulating and supporting a variety of organs in the body, including the digestive system, liver, and kidneys. It is a rich source of vitamins, minerals, and other nutrients that can help revitalize the body. Additionally, its diuretic properties support the elimination of toxins and excess fluid from the body. Dandelion is often used to support overall health and wellness.

- Dandelion is believed to support the health of the liver by promoting bile production, which aids in digestion and the absorption of nutrients.
- Dandelion also improves digestive health by increasing the production of stomach acid, promoting the growth of healthy gut bacteria, and reducing inflammation.
- Dandelion's antioxidants, vitamins, and minerals support a healthy immune system and protect the body from free radical damage.
- Dandelion's anti-inflammatory properties may reduce skin irritation and promote healthy skin. The compounds have also been shown to have anti-inflammatory effects throughout the body.
- Dandelion may help to regulate blood sugar levels by improving insulin sensitivity and reducing the absorption of glucose in the intestines.

Dandelion Root Decoction Recipe:

- Bring 2 cups of water to a boil, then reduce to a simmer.
- Add 2 teaspoons of dandelion root to the simmering water, then cover.
- Let it simmer for about 20 minutes.
- Strain the root.
- Add honey and lemon to taste if desired.
- Drink 1–2 mugs a day as needed.

Dandelion Tincture Recipe:

- Add fresh or dried dandelion root to a glass jar.
- Pour in enough alcohol to cover, leaving space at the top.*
- Tightly seal the jar, label, date, and shake well.
- Let it steep for 2–3 months. Shake the jar weekly.
- Strain the mixture, then store it in a glass jar in a dark place.
- Take 10–20 drops diluted in a little bit of water up to three times per day as needed.

- For children, the proper amount will vary depending on their age and weight. Use 5–7 drops diluted in a small amount of juice or water up to three times a day as needed.

Note: Dandelion is considered a gentle and safe tonic herb that can be used to support overall health and wellness. However, some people may experience allergic reactions to plants in the daisy family, such as ragweed and chrysanthemums. In addition, dandelion may be contraindicated with certain medications such as diuretics, blood thinners, and medications that are broken down by the liver. Always consult with a clinical herbalist or health care professional before taking herbal remedies, particularly if you have a health-related condition or are taking medication.

Licorice (Glycyrrhiza glabra)

Licorice is an adaptogen that works as a tonic herb in several ways. It contains glycyrrhizin, a compound with anti-inflammatory, anti-viral, and immune-boosting properties, as well as flavonoids and saponins that have antioxidant actions and protect the cells from damage caused by free radicals. Licorice helps the body cope with stress by supporting the adrenal glands and regulating cortisol levels.

As a tonic, licorice is believed to support the digestive system, soothe the respiratory tract, promote healthy skin, and support the immune system. It is used in traditional herbal medicine as a remedy for ulcers, coughs, colds, and fatigue.

Licorice Infusion Recipe:

- Bring 1 ½ cups of water to a boil, then reduce to a simmer.
- Add 1 teaspoon of licorice root to the simmering water, then cover.
- Simmer for 5–10 minutes.
- Strain the tea.
- Add lemon if desired.
- Drink 1–2 cups a day as needed.

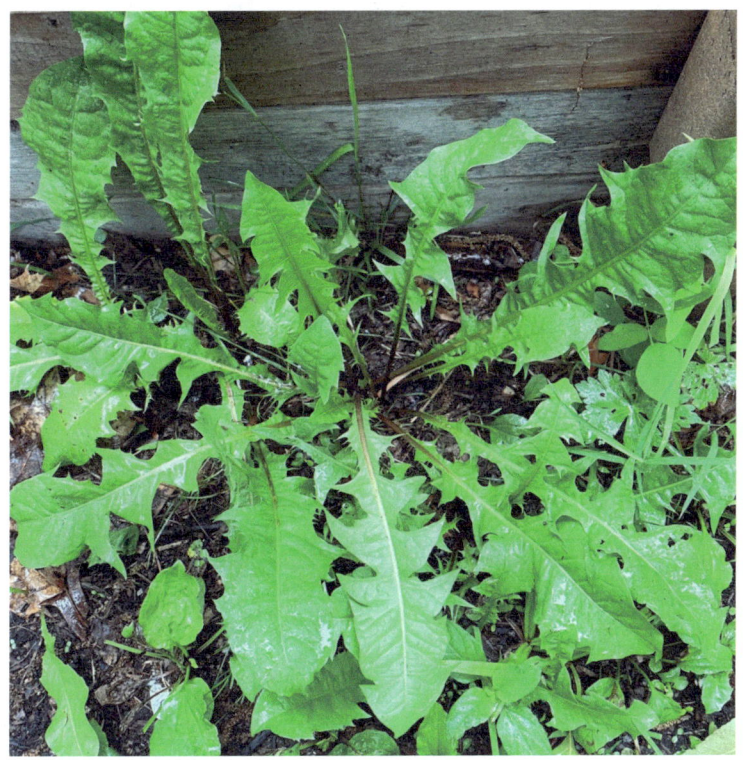

Note: Excessive consumption of licorice can have adverse effects. It may also have contraindications with certain medications. Always consult with a clinical herbalist or health care professional before taking herbal remedies, particularly if you have a health-related condition or are taking medication.

Elecampane (Inula helenium)

Elecampane is an adaptogen that is considered a tonic herb because it contains a variety of bioactive compounds, including sesquiterpene lactones, inulin, alantolactone, and isoalantolactone, that have beneficial effects on the body when taken over a period of time. These compounds are known for their anti-inflammatory, antioxidant, and antimicrobial properties that support overall health during a cold, flu, or viral infection. Rich in vitamins and minerals such as vitamins

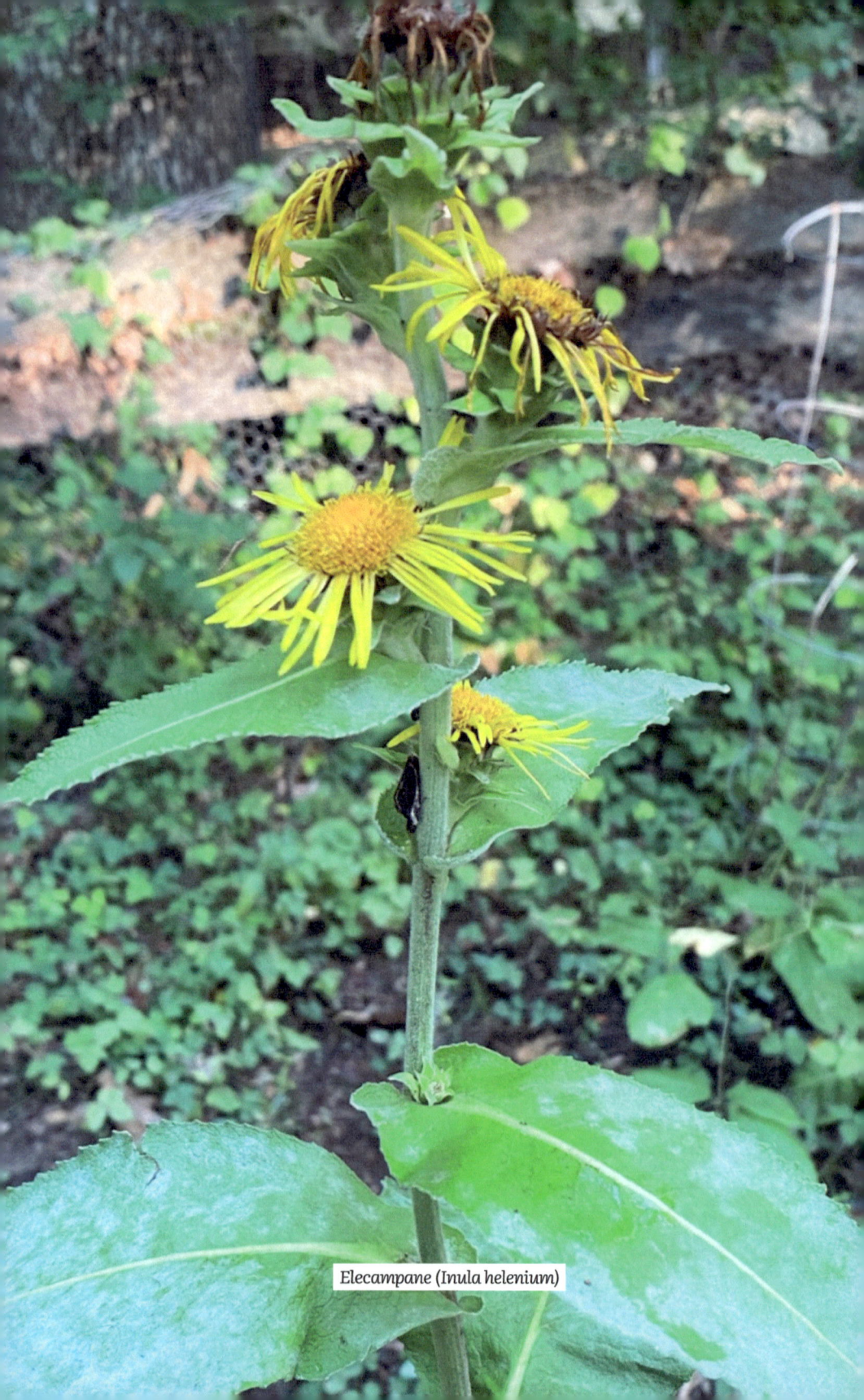
Elecampane (Inula helenium)

C and E, magnesium, potassium, and calcium, elecampane is a nourishing herb that supports the body's natural functions.

Elecampane Decoction Recipe:

- Bring 2 cups of water to a boil, then reduce to a simmer.
- Add 2 teaspoons of dried elecampane root to the pot, then cover.
- Simmer for 5–10 minutes.
- Strain the mixture.
- Add honey or lemon if desired.
- Drink 1–2 cups per day as needed. Elecampane is bitter, so drink slowly (an ounce or two at a time).

Elecampane Tincture Recipe:

- Fill a glass jar with chopped fresh or dried elecampane root.
- Pour in enough alcohol to cover, leaving space at the top.*
- Tightly seal the jar, label, date, and shake well.
- Let it steep for 2–3 months. Shake the jar weekly.
- Strain the tincture through cheesecloth or a fine mesh strainer.
- Store the tincture in a glass jar in a dark place.
- Take 15 drops diluted in a small amount of water or juice up to three times per day as needed.
- For children, the proper amount will vary depending on their age and weight. Use 5–7 drops diluted in a small amount of juice or water up to three times a day as needed.

Note: Elecampane should not be used during pregnancy or by individuals with a history of allergies to plants in the Asteraceae family. Always consult with a clinical herbalist or health care professional before taking herbal remedies, particularly if you have a health-related condition or are taking medication.

Coltsfoot (Tussilago farfara)

Coltsfoot, often considered a tonic, is an adaptogen herb due to its nutrient content. It contains potassium, magnesium, calcium, and vitamins A and C in addition to beneficial compounds such as mucilage, tannins, and flavonoids that amplify its health benefits. The mucilage in coltsfoot can help soothe and protect mucous membranes, while the tannins and flavonoids have anti-inflammatory and antioxidant properties.

Overall, coltsfoot is thought to have many nourishing and restorative effects, making it a useful tonic herb for supporting overall health and well-being.

Coltsfoot Infusion Recipe:

- Put 2 teaspoons of dried coltsfoot leaves and flowers in a tea ball or tea bag.
- Place in a mug and pour simmering water over the coltsfoot.
- Steep for 5–10 minutes
- Strain the tea.
- Drink 1–2 cups per day as needed.

Coltsfoot Tincture Recipe:

- Fill a glass jar with dried coltsfoot leaves and flowers.
- Pour in enough alcohol to cover, leaving space at the top.*
- Tightly seal the jar, label, date, and shake well.
- Let it steep for 2–3 months. Shake the jar weekly.
- Strain and store in a glass jar in a dark place.
- Take 3–5 drops diluted in a little bit of water up to twice a day as needed.
- Coltsfoot tincture is not recommended for children.

Note: Coltsfoot contains pyrrolizidine alkaloids, which have been shown to be toxic to the liver for some people if taken in large quantities or for prolonged periods of time. Always consult with a clinical herbalist or health care professional before taking herbal remedies, particularly if you have a health-related condition or are taking medication.

White Tea & Green Tea (Camellia sinensis)

White tea and green tea are both adaptogens considered to be tonic herbs. The primary active constituents of white and green tea leaves are polyphenols—specifically catechins—that act as potent antioxidants. Polyphenols help protect the body against free radical damage and inflammation linked to chronic diseases such as heart disease and diabetes. It also has the potential to support brain function and weight management.

White tea contains very little caffeine, but green tea has a considerably greater amount, giving it a stimulating effect on the central nervous system that can improve cognitive function and mental alertness. The theanine in white tea, on the other hand, has a calming effect on the central nervous system and can help reduce stress and anxiety. In addition, both teas contain other nutrients and compounds that can support overall health.

Note: Milk and non-dairy milk do not block the active constituents in white tea and green tea. However, adding milk to tea may decrease the absorption of certain antioxidants and polyphenols in the tea. This effect may be due to the proteins in the milk binding to the polyphenols and preventing them from being absorbed in the gut. To maximize the health benefits, it is recommended to drink white and green tea without adding milk.

White Tea Infusion Recipe:

- Put 2 teaspoons of dried white tea leaves in a tea ball or a tea bag.
- Place in a mug and pour simmering water over the tea.
- Steep for 3–5 minutes.
- Serve hot or cold with honey and lemon if desired.

White Tea Spritzer Recipe:

- Prepare white tea and let it cool in the refrigerator.
- To a glass, add ice, sparkling water, white tea, and a slice of lemon or lime.

Green Infusion Recipe:

- Put 2 teaspoons of dried green tea leaves in a tea ball or a tea bag.
- Place in a mug and pour simmering water over the tea.
- Steep for 2–3 minutes.
- Serve hot or cold with honey and lemon if desired.

Matcha Latte Recipe:

- Whisk 1 teaspoon of matcha powder with 2 ounces of simmering water until frothy.
- Add 1 cup of steamed milk and honey or maple syrup to taste.

Green Tea Smoothie Recipe:

- In a blender, combine 1 teaspoon of green tea leaves, 1 cup of fresh or frozen kale, 1 frozen banana, 1 cup of aromatic herb tea (such as peppermint or lemon balm tea), and 1 tablespoon of honey or maple syrup.
- Whiz until smooth.

Tonic Foods and Recipes

Bone Broth:

- Simmer bones (chicken, beef, or fish) in a pot of water for several hours. Try a variety of vegetables, herbs, and spices for different flavors.

Bone broth is rich in gelatin and nutrients such as collagen, calcium, magnesium, and phosphorus that support the immune system and overall health.

Green Smoothie:

- Blend together fresh or frozen spinach or avocado, banana, ginger, and aromatic tea for a nutritious, mineral-rich, and tasty smoothie.

Chia Seed Pudding:

- Mix chia seeds with non-dairy milk, honey, and vanilla extract and let it sit in the refrigerator overnight for a nutritious and delicious pudding.

Chia seeds are rich in omega-3s, fiber, and protein.

Miso Soup:

- Combine miso paste with simmering water. Do not boil—the intense heat will kill the probiotics.
- Add seaweed, tofu, and green onions to taste.

Miso is a fermented soybean paste rich in probiotics and other beneficial nutrients.

Turmeric Tea:

- Boil water with turmeric powder, ginger, and honey for a soothing and healing drink.

Turmeric is a powerful anti-inflammatory spice that is great for overall health.

Fermented Foods:

Sauerkraut, kimchi, kefir, and yogurt are all great sources of probiotics that support the microbiome and the growth of good bacterium for a healthy gut and overall health.

Oatmeal:

- Prepare oats and add yogurt, fruits, nuts, yogurt, maple syrup, and spices such as cinnamon for a tasty and nutritious breakfast.

Oatmeal is nutrient rich and fibrous food that is healthy for the digestive system.

Berries:

Berries such as raspberries, blackberries, blueberries, and strawberries are rich in antioxidants and other beneficial nutrients that support overall health. You can add them to smoothies, yogurt, or eat them as a snack.

Nuts and Seeds:

Almonds, walnuts, sunflower seeds, pumpkin seeds, and chia seeds are great sources of healthy fats, protein, and other beneficial nutrients. You can add them to salads, oatmeal, or eat them as a snack.

Dark Leafy Greens:

Kale, spinach, parsley, and collard greens are rich in vitamins, minerals, and antioxidants that support overall health. These greens can be added to smoothies, eaten in salads, or sautéed.

Miso Soup with Vegetables and Bone Broth

Ingredients:

- 4 cups beef or chicken bone broth
- 1 cup chopped or sliced shiitake mushrooms
- 1 cup chopped or sliced bok choy or celery
- ½ cup onions, sliced or minced
- 2 garlic cloves, minced
- 1 tbsp ginger, grated
- 1 tbsp red or white miso paste
- 1 tbsp extra virgin olive oil

- 1 tbsp tamari or Braggs liquid aminos
- 1 tbsp of rice or apple cider vinegar
- Salt and pepper to taste

Add more vegetables of your choice for additional nutrients and flavor.

Instructions:

- Heat the extra virgin olive oil in a pot over medium heat.
- Add onions and garlic and sauté until fragrant.
- Add shiitake mushrooms and celery or bok choy to the pot and cook until tender.
- Add bone broth, ginger, tamari or Braggs, and vinegar to the pot and bring to a boil.
- Turn down the heat and let the soup simmer for 10 minutes.
- In a separate bowl, combine miso paste with a ladle of the broth and mix until the miso dissolves.
- Add the miso mixture to the pot and stir well. Do not boil, as the heat will kill the beneficial bacteria in the miso.
- Add salt and pepper to taste.
- Serve hot and enjoy this comforting and nourishing soup.

A berry, Nut, and Seed Dessert:

Ingredients:

- 2 cups mixed berries
- ½ cup chopped mixed nuts
- ¼ cup mixed seeds
- 1 tablespoon honey (optional)
- ¼ teaspoon cinnamon (optional)

vInstructions:

- Preheat your oven to 350°F.
- Spread the chopped nuts and seeds in a single layer on a baking sheet and toast in the oven for 8–10 minutes, until lightly browned and fragrant. Set aside to cool.
- Divide the berries evenly among four dessert bowls or glasses.
- Sprinkle the roasted nuts and seeds over the berries.
- Drizzle the honey over the top.
- Sprinkle with cinnamon.
- Enjoy warm fresh out of the oven.

A Berry, Nut, Seed, and Yogurt Parfait:

Ingredients:

- 1 cup mixed berries
- ¼ cup chopped nuts
- ¼ cup mixed seeds
- 1 cup plain Greek yogurt
- 1 tablespoon honey (optional)

Instructions:

- In a small bowl, mix the chopped nuts and mixed seeds.
- Layer the berries, the nut and seed mixture, and yogurt in a serving bowl or glass.
- Repeat until all the ingredients are used up.
- Drizzle with honey if desired.

CONCLUSION

Whole foods and herbal remedies provide a wide range of health benefits and actions to support our holistic constitution. Combining the power of whole foods with herbal remedies can support and strengthen our immune systems and help fight off colds, flus, viruses, and viral infections without throwing the body's homeostasis out of balance.

Many of the herbs and foods I have included in this book fit into more than one category of herbal actions. This pattern is designed to show the value of whole plants' affinity to our holistic system. Herbal affinity is of a higher intelligence; it is designed to stay one step ahead of the holistic system to nurture and strengthen the body's condition. To block and stop a virus or to wipe it out completely prevents that illness from worsening or becoming a chronic condition, causing more serious disease that would weaken our homeostasis and our holistic system. Whole foods nurture, energize, and cleanse the body. Eating the right foods to support the effects of the herbal remedies further strengthens our immune system, giving it every opportunity to wipe out infections and protect us from a more serious disease.

Our body must endure to fight a viral infection. Our body, mind, and spirit should all be aligned to promote health and balance for our homeostasis. Homeostasis is the maintenance of a stable and balanced internal environment in the body despite external changes. It involves a complex system of processes that work together to regulate and balance various physiological functions, including our body's temperature, blood pressure, pH levels, fluid and electrolyte balance, and hormone levels. Homeostasis is crucial for the body's proper functioning, and disruptions to homeostasis can lead to various health problems. In holistic health, homeostasis is viewed as an essential aspect of overall well-being, which includes our physical, emotional, mental, health, and spiritual well-being.

We are like a ship at sea. Our focus, balance, and spirit should be calm when we are being tossed to and fro while fighting an illness. Being able to consciously draw your attention to your spirit, the center of your whole being, should help you remain calm and ride out the storm. Start to observe love in spirit form. Pull on love, draw it in. Cherish it. Talk to it. Let it enlighten you. I see colors in my mind's eye. My journey begins anew every moment I can reflect on love.

Sometimes, I feel impure when the virus is flaring and starting to blaze; when I am weak, my focus and emotions spiral downward. I speak to it, address it, identify it, and acknowledge, greater is He that is in me than He who is in this world. No weapon formed against me shall prosper. Shine light on it. Chase the darkness away through every channel you know. Believe what you are speaking, as the power of words or your prayers may purify your thoughts, your body's illness, and bring peace to your soul.

Herbs and whole foods need our commitment to fulfill their purpose and support our wellbeing. We must align to strengthen our defenses. Where two or more are joined, there is the presence of love. Whole foods and herbs work synergistically to help us recover and stay healthy. Love yourself so you can embrace love, bring it in, speak to it, admire it, and know its glory—it is the light of the world. The only thing left untouched to complete your self-care is a little encouragement. Show gratitude for the air you breathe. Live in love and with love through it all to calm the storm.

Breathe in light, breathe out darkness.

Be healed,

Anna Sangemino

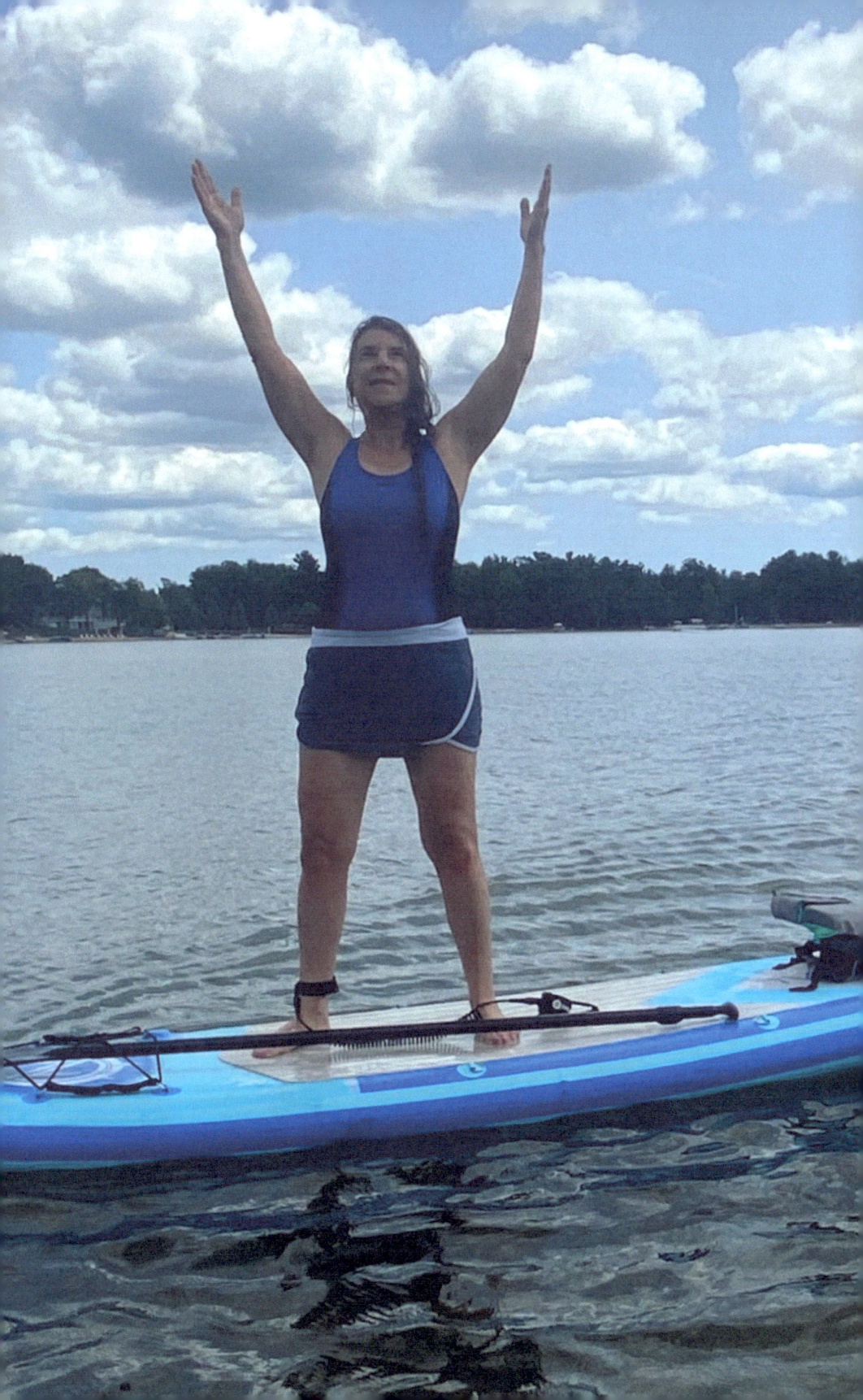

Made in the USA
Columbia, SC
29 September 2024